Pelican Books
The Safety of the Unborn Child

Geoffrey Chamberlain was born in Sussex in 1930. He was at
school in Cowbridge during the war, and qualified as a
doctor from University College Hospital, London, in 1954.
Since then he has practised medicine in England and
America. Being a busy practical obstetrician at a London
teaching hospital, he has learnt his subject by teaching it, not
only to medical students and doctors, but also to his
patients.

Mr Chamberlain has published many articles on research
and clinical obstetrics in medical journals on both sides of
the Atlantic. In 1966, as the Thomas Eden fellow of the
Royal College of Obstetricians and Gynaecologists, he spent
a year in Washington, U.S.A., doing research into problems
of premature babies. He was there awarded the annual
Foundation prize of the American Association of
Obstetricians and Gynaecologists for this work. He is now
permanently back in this country.

Geoffrey Chamberlain

The Safety of the
Unborn Child

Penguin Books

Penguin Books Ltd, Harmondsworth,
Middlesex, England
Penguin Books Inc., 7110 Ambassador Road,
Baltimore, Maryland 21207, U.S.A.
Penguin Books Australia Ltd, Ringwood,
Victoria, Australia

First published 1969
Copyright © Geoffrey Chamberlain, 1969

Made and printed in Great Britain by
C. Nicholls & Company Ltd
Set in Linotype Times

Contents

Foreword

We are often reminded that a little knowledge is a dangerous thing, but less often that ignorance is equally dangerous and ignorance in action often calamitous. We live in a society where, although there are still some who prefer to live in an ivory tower of intellectual seclusion, and some who are content to live with their heads in the sand, there is an ever-increasing number of those who want to be informed. As the general levels of understanding and education improve, it is inevitable that the articulate and intelligent members of society will want to know more about medical problems as and when they are themselves affected by them. Because of built-in traditional objection to any form of publicity by the medical profession, and perhaps some apprehension about the possibilities of disciplinary action, we have, as a profession, been slow to communicate with the public *en masse*, however well we communicate across the consultation desk. The situation has therefore arisen that much of the communication has been taken over by mass media – newspapers, magazines, radio, television – and those who communicate are all too often lay men and women, who, however much trouble and time they may take to inform themselves, still remain ill-equipped for their task. Sensationalism and news value often take precedence over scientific accuracy, and so the public are often misinformed and misled.

In modern society, therefore, the doctor must more and more enter the field of education of the laity, and there is no better time in which to attempt the education of the female members of society than during the ante-natal and post-natal periods. At these times women are intensely interested in

Foreword

what goes on, and excited at the prospect of reproducing another life. They are receptive to ideas and willing to do all sorts of things they might otherwise resent, because they are being done for someone else as well as for themselves. The need to communicate is paramount in good medical practice, and the doctor loses nothing of his prestige and stature by explaining facts in simple language that the layman can understand.

To write a book for the lay public on obstetrics is no mean undertaking. Mr Chamberlain is to be congratulated on even contemplating the possibility of so doing – and the achievement is even more to be commended. The theme of the book is the unborn child, what happens to it as it grows and develops, and what events occurring during pregnancy may adversely affect its normal progress. This book goes far beyond the many books already in existence on ante-natal care and advice to the mother, and so it will appeal only to the more intelligent reader. Nevertheless, it is eminently readable, written in a flowing style which makes one feel that the author is actually talking to the patient; this fact I am sure will be appreciated by those most likely to read it.

I commend it as a challenging experiment; as a carefully planned and well-produced volume, provided with a glossary of definitions and explanations of terms in common use which will be found most helpful.

Sir John Peel, President,
Royal College of Obstetricians and Gynaecologists
Regent's Park, London N.W.1.

Preface

This book is written to answer many of the questions the pregnant woman asks about her unborn child. This infant is causing a major alteration in her life, and it is right that he should occupy her thoughts.

While investigating the attitudes of pregnant women to pre-natal instruction and education, we asked a number of patients attending ante-natal clinics to fill in an anonymous questionnaire. One patient wrote of the doctor's reaction to answering questions about pregnancy: 'I feel that there is an atmosphere of "No need to tell them what's going on – they won't understand." This isn't true. Most mothers-to-be are very much interested in their condition and want all the facts explained.' This patient's thoughts were echoed in the rest of the survey; 59 per cent of those having their first baby were attending instruction, while 78 per cent of all the mothers were reading books about pregnancy.

In spite of the apparent hurry and bustle that often attends an ante-natal clinic, it is the hope of the medical staff that they deal adequately with the natural doubts and worries of the pregnant woman. Obviously some patients voice their thoughts more easily than others, and it is from these that we learn of commonly recurrent fears. The rest may not ask, and for them this book is written, in the hope that it may deal with some of the points which have secretly disturbed them.

To condense our knowledge of pregnancy into one small volume has obviously necessitated much compression, and in many sections I have been dogmatic. Doctors are humans looking after other humans, and opinion must enter into every decision they make. However, all the observations in the text have either been made personally or have been quoted from articles published in medical journals, and I should like to acknowledge my indebtedness to the many researchers in

9

Preface

Great Britain and America whose work I have quoted. Especially I should like to thank the consultant staff of King's College Hospital and the British Hospital for Mothers and Babies in Woolwich for allowing me to work with their patients. Many others have helped by providing information in their own special fields, and I am most grateful to Professor R. W. Smithells of the Alder Hay Hospital in Liverpool. He as one of the first workers on the causation of congenital defects, has been a constant stimulus and source of help to others in this field.

To illustrate the book I have been fortunate in obtaining material from other obstetrical departments. For their help in this matter I should like to thank Professor Ian Donald of Glasgow for his Sonar illustration (Plate 7), Professor Philip Rhodes of St Thomas's Hospital for the illustration of the uterine blood supply (Plate 10), Dr Charles Whitfield of Belfast for his foetal electrocardiograph tracing (Figure 15) and Professor W. Davidson of my own hospital, who lent the chromosome pictures and their karyometric classification (Plates 8 and 9). Many of the photographs were taken by Mr W. Smith of King's College Hospital Photographic Department, to whom I am most grateful.

The first part of the book gives an idea of the incidents occurring in any pregnancy. An outline of the ante-natal clinic routine is shown, and an explanation provided of the tests performed. The problems dealt with in the second two sections are those which pregnant women may come across or think about, and the chapters are based upon the thoughts and worries expressed by a large number of patients. Here the mother will find answers to many of her questions about the welfare of her unborn child. It is hoped that the knowledge gained will help the pregnancy to pass more happily and that, so forearmed, the patient will find herself approaching the baby's birth more easily. She will realize that nearly every child is normal and will stay so; that nearly every labour is uncomplicated and produces a worthwhile result.

Geoffrey Chamberlain M.D., F.R.C.S., M.R.C.O.G.
Forest Hill, London S.E., 1968

1 | The Intra-uterine State

1 | Ante-natal Care

In the nineteenth century, the medical profession reflected one aspect of the hierarchical state of society. The right of the rich and educated to dictate to the poor and ignorant was virtually unchallenged; it was felt that the lower social orders were incapable of profiting from education, which was therefore denied them. In this situation knowledge meant power, and remained firmly in the hands of the professions and upper classes. This principle of keeping knowledge from the ignorant was carried over by doctors to their treatment of women in childbirth; they hid the principles of medicine, ill-understood though they were, and considered it wrong, if not actually dangerous, for a woman to know about her unborn baby or the process of his growth. Such prejudices were reinforced by the large folklore which has always surrounded childbirth. Gossip and exaggeration bred tales which would frighten the strongest of us. Modern versions of these superstitions are still bandied around and may be heard in the queues waiting at ante-natal clinics. Some are cruel, most are groundless, and all are based on exaggerated, ill-conceived ideas of what goes on in pregnancy and labour.

Gradually, it was realized that the best way to overcome the fears engendered by the horror stories was to let women know something of the truth. The unknown is always more frightening than the known, and now, in the middle of the twentieth century, most doctors prefer that their patients should have some idea about what is happening to them.

13

The Intra-uterine State

We try to prepare expectant mothers, so that they come to labour with a knowledge of forthcoming events; these women have more understanding and so are more cooperative in both mind and body.

Ante-natal Instruction

Ante-natal instruction is not an easy business, for in this situation it is more important for patients to understand the facts than to learn them. The first does not always follow the second. Teaching students the irregular verbs in French is easier than helping them to understand the philosophy of Voltaire. For a pupil to gain understanding he should ideally be taught by an individual instructor, and the speed of instruction should be varied. In ante-natal instruction, however, the classes of mothers to whom the doctor must explain the details of pregnancy and labour are often large. He directs his teaching to the average mother and, while some of his hearers cannot keep pace with him, others rapidly understand what he is saying and the rest of the ante-natal instruction time is wasted for them. It is here that individual tuition would be excellent if it were available, for during pregnancy the mother's mind naturally dwells on forthcoming events, and women react in different ways to the whole strange concept of a living baby being inside them. Some accept this fact early and, taking the hopeful view that everything will go normally, are eager to learn more about the process. For others the major pre-occupation is that the child may not be normal or may even be born dead. This seems to be the natural reaction of many women, even those who are well-balanced, and it is perhaps especially towards these readers that this book is directed.

Perhaps most mothers dread deformity for their forth-coming infants even more than death. Many women reason that, although death causes pain, it is at least over quickly and the sorrow is to a greater or lesser degree healed by time. The malformed child, however, remains with the family and is a constant reminder of grief. In addition to this, the days are not long past when the birth of such an infant was considered to be an act of God, a punishment for sins committed. Nowadays there is a much less cen-sorious theological attitude, but still the unconscious mind sometimes betrays us. Many women, even if they have com-mitted no major sins, can find some acts of which they are ashamed if they search their memories deeply, and the shock of producing a less than perfect infant is enough to bring unconscious fears to the surface. There is no evidence, however, that pregnancies are affected by past behaviour.

An essential part of ante-natal care should consist of seeking out and dealing with such thoughts. At present many ante-natal organizations run classes and discussion groups. These are good in that they give instruction. How-ever, they do not go far enough, for some women may not like to ask questions in front of others. They may think their questions will sound elementary and silly, and they may also be timid in exposing what seem groundless fears. These problems may be elementary, but they are certainly not silly. Any problem that is worrying a mother should be expressed openly and should be answered.

Both for giving information and for allaying fear, then, groups and classes are unsatisfactory. The ideal is indivi-dual instruction, but in Great Britain at present this indivi-dual attention is given only in private practice, or to those who attend their own general practitioner for their ante-natal welfare. Three quarters of the women in this country attend large, impersonal hospital or local authority clinics. These provide good medical diagnostic care, but are too impersonal for the patients to get to know the doctors. At many first-class hospitals running National Health Service obstetric units, mothers attending the ante-natal clinic see, on average, five different doctors at various stages in their ante-natal care. This is due to changes of staff and organization of duty rotas. Rapport is difficult to establish, and most women do not like putting questions to a comparative stranger.

When a patient is on the couch at an ante-natal clinic, the doctors seeing her can use this opportunity to answer any queries she may have. The material of this book is derived from the questions that have been asked at such sessions. Recently the author looked after an intelligent patient who had taken a good first-class degree at one of the older universities. She was tense and anxious, and no amount of discussion in the brief time allowed in the hospital clinic could alleviate this. Finally, after a normal delivery, she explained the problem. She had read of 'Bloody Mary', Queen of England, who was alleged to have had a twenty-month pregnancy. Although the patient knew that most women delivered themselves in nine months, she was afraid lest she, like Mary, was an exception and might continue to be pregnant for almost two years. This was a misunderstanding that could have been corrected easily had she ever brought herself to talk freely. There is no truth in the tale about Queen Mary; in fact she was never pregnant. The problem seemed too silly for our patient to mention to any of us, and so it festered in her mind.

From patients like this one, we learn of the mass of questions which pregnant women would like to ask. This book tries to answer some of them. Being a book it can be picked up and put down. Parts can be re-read until they are clear; other parts can be skipped. Further, it may help patients to phrase their questions to their own medical attendants so that answers to their individual difficulties can be obtained.

Ante-natal Surveillance

In Great Britain about two thirds of babies are born in hospital or nursing homes. More would be so delivered, but because of the deficiencies of the National Health Service the country is short of maternity beds. Not all mothers wishing for a hospital confinement can be accommodated. A few women energetically desire home confinement, and those suitable are usually safely delivered by their general practitioners; but the majority of mothers ask for hospital beds. Usually those women to whom beds are allocated receive their ante-natal care at the hospital which is looking after them, although a few may go to their own family doctor where he is in a cooperative scheme with the hospital. Those who are to be delivered at home receive their care either from their general practitioner or from a local authority ante-natal clinic. Wherever the patients go – hospital, family doctor or local authority clinic – the standards of ante-natal care are good in Britain; obstetrics is preventive medicine, ensuring that things do not go wrong, and detecting untoward happenings at an early stage, when it is easier to correct them.

First Clinic Visit

Most patients go to their doctor when they first suspect pregnancy. This is generally about four to eight weeks after the first missed period. The diagnosis having been confirmed, the patient is referred to those who will look after her in pregnancy and labour. The first visit to the ante-natal clinic therefore comes at about twelve weeks of pregnancy. The patient is usually welcomed by a midwife, who requests some information about her past medical care. Details of past illnesses and operations are recorded, for these may influence the progress of pregnancy. Her family history is inquired after, and she is asked about present living conditions. When this is not the first baby, details of previous pregnancies and births are also recorded. Sometimes the mother may not know all the relevant details, and in that case the information is obtained from any hospital in which a previous birth took place. The events of this present pregnancy are taken down. The importance of the date of the last menstrual period is stressed in the next chapter.

The patient's weight and height are then usually recorded. The former should be known so that at subsequent visits the weight-gain in pregnancy can be checked. The patient's height may be a guide to the doctor in assessing the size of her bony pelvis and so of the passage through which the baby must pass in labour. The mother is then seen by the doctor at the clinic, who will usually check those points of the past medical history that might be considered important. Next, a full medical examination is performed. Included in this is an assessment of the heart and lungs by examination of the chest, and measurement of the blood pressure. The patient's teeth are examined, and if there is any doubt as to their condition she is advised to consult her dentist. (Under the National Health Service, dental care in Great Britain is free for pregnant women.) Any dental degeneration may progress rapidly at this time because the increased production of cortisone, stimulated by the pregnancy, is liable to speed the progress of any inflammation of the teeth or gums. Further, the growing baby in the uterus demands a large amount of calcium salts to strengthen his growing bones. These can come only from the mother, and unless her diet contains an increase of calcium substances it is her stores that will be depleted to provide for the baby. The teeth are one of the parts of her body where calcium is richly laid down, and in pregnancy they may be irreparably denuded of their strength if the baby's demand for calcium is drawn mainly from them, so that caries is allowed to take hold.

Examination of the abdomen by the doctor may show that the uterus is enlarged. By about the twelfth to fourteenth week of pregnancy, the uterus and the embryo it contains have grown enough to fill the pelvis and rise into the general abdominal cavity, so that they can be felt by the examining hand (see Figure 1). During this examination,

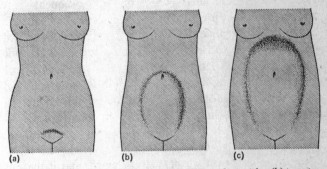

Figure 1. The size of the growing uterus at (a) twelve weeks, (b) twenty-four weeks, and (c) thirty-six weeks of pregnancy.

the doctor will be on the look-out for any enlargements of other abdominal organs.

Many doctors next perform a pelvic examination,

19

though others postpone this to a later date. Some women build up an unpleasant imaginary picture of this part of the visit to the clinic, making themselves nervous about it and often spreading alarm to others. A pelvic examination (vaginal or internal examination) does not hurt. The doctor's finger is passed into the vagina, and the pelvic organs are palpated between the doctor's two hands, the one steadying the neck of the womb in the vagina, the other moving on the surface of the abdomen (see Figure 2). No

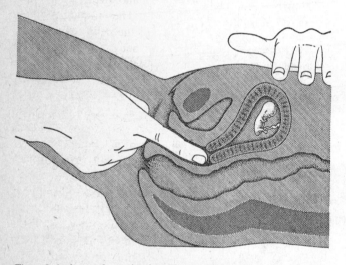

Figure 2. An internal examination. The condition of the pelvic organs is thoroughly assessed by the doctor's hands.

one would pretend that such an examination is pleasant, but it is usually not even uncomfortable and certainly not painful. But if the patient has allowed her fears to build up in her mind, the muscles that surround the vagina may go into spasm. They become tight and hard and prevent the examining finger from doing its job. This spasm may indeed be painful but it is engineered in the patient's own mind, and not caused by the doctor's finger.

The internal examination is essential for the welfare of the mother, and for her baby's safety. Sometimes, patients attend the ante-natal clinic before the uterus has grown enough to be felt by palpation of the abdomen only. The internal examination enables lesser enlargements to be assessed and accurately recorded. Any abnormalities in the shape of the uterus can be judged, and at the same time a check can be made on the ovaries. The internal examination also allows an investigation of the pelvis to be made. The parts shaded in Figure 2 are bony, and through this bony canal the baby has to pass in labour. At this early stage, the doctor can assess the birth canal and its ability to accommodate the baby. Few women would buy a dress for a child without first checking that it fitted. How much more important is this preliminary examination to check that the mother's pelvis will fit the baby in labour!

At this time, a sample of blood is usually taken from a vein in the patient's forearm. Only a small amount is withdrawn, and the body, which contains eight to ten pints, does not miss it. This sample is examined in the laboratory, where the mother's blood groups are determined, and the blood is checked for anaemia. It is important for the welfare of both mother and child to know the blood groups well before birth. Certain diseases (for example, syphilis) could leave their signs in the blood and tests can be made for them. All these investigations give the doctors further information about the patient and her developing pregnancy, and they allow special treatment to be used if necessary.

In many cases, the ante-natal clinic provides a patient's

first full medical check since she left school. Occasionally some symptom-free disability is detected, and this can then be treated early. On the whole, patients of the age-group attending ante-natal clinics are fit and well, but one condition still has to be looked for: tuberculosis. This disease is on the decrease – largely owing to the routine mass miniature chest X-ray examination, popularized just before and during the Second World War. In ante-natal clinics we still occasionally see patients with incipient tuberculosis, which can easily be treated and completely cured. Pregnancy can exacerbate this disease, and so a chest X-ray is a wise precaution in the early stages of any pregnancy, and it is usually arranged at the first visit to the clinic. Those taking the chest X-ray are well aware of the existence of the pregnancy and take screening precautions with lead shields to protect the embryo (see Plate 1).

This usually concludes the first visit to the clinic. It is the most thorough (and the longest) visit; it gives the doctors who will look after the mother a comprehensive idea of her health and of her capacity to deliver herself of a healthy baby at the end of the pregnancy.

Other Ante-natal Visits

The mother leaves the first clinic clutching a box of iron tablets, and with her certificate of expected confinement, a booklet or two on ante-natal welfare, a mind full of impressions, and an appointment to return in a month. The first few can be dealt with by being eaten, posted, read and mentally digested, but the last often remains a bit of a mystery. Why do doctors want to see their patients at intervals in pregnancy? Surely they have probed and learnt enough at the exhaustive first visit to the clinic? There can be little left to find out.

Pregnancy is not a static process; it is a dynamic one, constantly altering as the embryo grows into a baby, and the mother's body changes in its relationship with that baby. These changes lead to variations in the mother's condition which need frequent observations. Further, the baby's progress and position should be assessed, for the approach to labour may need modifying if the situation becomes unfavourable. One of the commonest causes of infant and even maternal death, for instance, used to be toxaemia of pregnancy (pre-eclampsia). This has been considerably curtailed as a direct result of frequent regular checks on the mother's health.

Early in pregnancy a monthly visit is sufficient, but after thirty-two weeks a fortnightly attendance is more usual. From the thirty-sixth week, most patients come to the clinic weekly. At all these visits the patient's health is checked. Her blood pressure is measured and her urine tested. (Do be sure that the sample of the latter is in a clean bottle. Not long ago an epidemic of sugar diabetes was thought to have occurred among pregnant women at one London hospital. All the mothers had been using concentrated orange juice bottles for their samples, and although they had been washed, it had been forgotten that the cardboard lining of the screw cap can absorb sugar-rich orange juice.) The patient's abdomen is examined, and the rate of growth of the uterus is checked. Late in pregnancy the developing baby can be felt through the uterine wall and usually the head and spine can be easily detected. (In the case of a thin mother with a thin-walled uterus the baby's limbs and even the fingers and toes can be felt.) The infant's heart can be heard beating inside the uterus from just after mid-pregnancy (approximately twenty-four to twenty-eight weeks). In the last six to eight weeks of pregnancy the infant usually settles to a head-down position. If he does not, many doctors encourage him to do so by manoeuvring him round by gentle pressure on the mother's abdominal wall at clinic visits. The last three weeks of the first pregnancy are often associated with the baby's head going down into the pelvis – the head is described as becoming 'engaged'. This means that the largest diameter of the baby's head has passed through the bony inlet of the pelvis. Once a baby's head (its largest part) has entered the pelvis, usually any doubts of that baby being too large for that mother's pelvis are removed. This point is carefully checked by the examining doctor. A sample of blood is often taken in the last ten weeks of pregnancy to check that the patient is not becoming anaemic. Sometimes, the blood-group estimation in early pregnancy warns of a potentially difficult situation in a few women of certain Rhesus blood groups (see Chapter 11). The progress of their infants may be assessed by checking the mother's blood in the later stages of the pregnancy.

Not all these procedures are gone through at each visit, but the basic checking of blood pressure and urine, and the abdominal examination, are done. This is the time that the patient should use to ask her doctor about points that may worry her. There may seem to be a big queue at the clinic, but there is always time to answer questions. At the author's hospital the ante-natal clinics are large. A recent survey showed that only 11 per cent of our patients found there was insufficient time to ask any questions, so presumably 89 per cent feel they can ask and receive answers to any questions that arise.

Ante-natal Lectures

Many clinics now provide a series of talks for mothers, usually given by senior midwives and medical staff. Their value varies greatly from one institution to the next. Obviously the enthusiasm and ability of those running these series are important. Generally the subject-matter deals with the usual progress of later pregnancy and labour. It often includes films of a baby's birth and, ideally, a tour of the delivery suite, to show what a labour ward looks like. All this instruction is usually aimed at getting the baby born, and little time is spent on the baby himself. Some hospitals hold talks for the father-to-be, but these too emphasize his supportive role to the wife in 'the difficult time to come', and do little to inform him about the offspring. Some women attend relaxation classes and talks about ante-natal exercises and breathing techniques. These are helpful to most women, but again no one gives any information about the source of so much of the mother's thinking – the baby.

Briefly this book tells of the unborn child's development from a fertilized egg to birth. Parts may be technical and can be skipped; other sections do not concern all pregnancies. Certain chapters, however, are of common interest to all pregnant women. The book also mentions the known ways in which development may go wrong. The author hopes that, by giving a true perspective, he can help mothers to realize that nearly every baby is in fact a normal one. Thus many groundless fears may be allayed before they become major problems, and the course of pregnancy and labour will be smoother.

2 | The Development of the Embryo

The proper understanding of a newborn baby must include some idea of how it grew. All human beings start from a single cell. This divides and develops to produce the complex body which includes many different organs and systems, all serving different functions. This chapter is a technical account of these processes.

Length of Pregnancy

From conception to delivery in the human is usually 266 days. Generally, in mammals (of which we are one species), the length of gestation bears a relation to the size of the body. Not all humans are exactly the same, but 90 per cent of women who are sure of the date of their last menstruation, and have a 28-day cycle, will deliver within 10 days of the date expected.

Most married women do not know the exact date of conception. Either intercourse has occurred several times, or the date of a single time is forgotten. So the convention has arisen of dating the duration of a pregnancy from the last menstrual period. A woman who has a 28-day cycle will ovulate, that is produce an egg-cell from one of her ovaries, about half-way between the periods. Pregnancy is thus considered to last 280 days from the first day of the last normal menstrual period (that is, 266 + 14 days). Obviously the woman is not pregnant for the first 14 days of this time for she has not yet ovulated, but the convention used is a convenient one.

280 days is exactly 40 weeks, and weeks are the units used by doctors in timing a pregnancy. Although women usually think in terms of months, this can lead to confusion, for 280 days (40 weeks) is ten 28-day lunar months or nine variable calendar months and one week. We rarely think in lunar months, and calendar months vary in length. (See the Chronological Table on page 176.)

Although 90 per cent of women are delivered reasonably close to the 280-day mark, some have their babies much earlier, and a few much later. The child who is born early will be smaller and less well developed. Such children are immature and not so well adapted to the stresses of life outside the uterus. They are clearly at higher risk than mature infants, and the hazards bear a strong relationship to the size of the child. However, many children born at two or three pounds live and thrive. The smallest baby known to survive, born in 1937 at South Shields, was sixteen ounces at birth; her family doctor kept her alive by hourly feeds with a fountain-pen filler, and she is now a healthy mother herself. Better facilities in premature-baby nurseries throughout the country are saving many more infants by the use of intensive nursing and medical care. Prematurity is discussed fully in Chapter 12.

Pregnancies that continue past their expected date do not produce proportionately larger infants. Growth is very much a factor of the healthy placenta; after full term is reached, this organ ages rapidly, and so growth rates slow down. The author has, however, delivered a baby of fifteen pounds, and even heavier ones are known. Two or three over twenty pounds have been recorded, but some of these were born by Caesarean section. Such large babies are rare, and in Britain 93 per cent of babies are born weighing less than ten pounds.

Ovulation and Conception

Between each menstrual period during reproductive life, a woman sheds an egg from one of her ovaries. This passes into the outer, open end of the Fallopian tube (see Figure

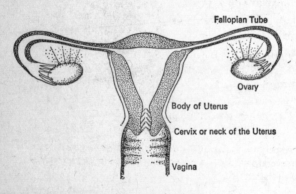

Figure 3. Female reproductive organs in section.

3). The egg has no means of active locomotion but is propelled by rhythmical contractions of the tube wall. Should intercourse have taken place within the past twenty-four hours, spermatozoa (which are active) will have swum up the canal of the cervix, through the uterine cavity and along the Fallopian tube. The sperm seems to be attracted to the egg by a chemical which the latter releases into the surrounding fluid; this is comparable with the fact that male moths swarm for miles after a female that they can smell. The sperm approaches the egg, its head pierces the outermost membrane and its nucleus then fuses with that of the egg (Figure 4). Once the egg is impregnated, the membranes become impermeable to any other sperm. Both the egg and the sperm carry in their nuclei genes from each parent which

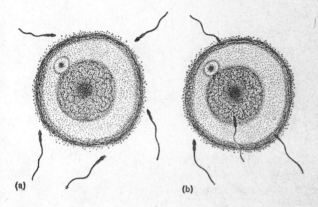

Figure 4. A sperm approaching (a) and fusing with (b) a human ovum. Although several have penetrated the outer layer, only one spermatozoon reaches the nucleus.

determine the future genetical make-up of the child; the fertilized egg has thus, from the earliest stage, the full hereditary background of both the mother and the father. Genes, and their place in the handing-on of characteristics, are more fully discussed in Chapter 6.

Early Development

Soon after fertilization, the single cell divides into two by the splitting first of its nucleus and then of the cell substance (see Figure 5). In the nucleus the genes carrying the inherited characteristics are also split, and equal amounts go to each

29

of the new cells. The two cells each then split to form a four-cell mass, and so, by repeated divisions, eight, sixteen and thirty-two cells in turn are formed. The nucleus of each cell carries a complete replica of all the genes and thus the full hereditary potential of the child.

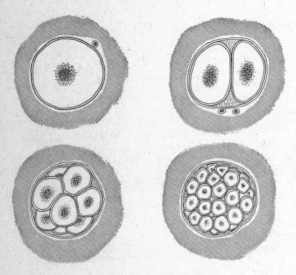

Figure 5. Cell division showing increase in cell mass. All cells contain the nucleal and chromosome material of the original cell.

Until the thirty-two-cell stage, the knot of cells is compact and all cells have some part of their surface in contact with the outside world. Through this surface all the oxygen necessary for life and growth is obtained by diffusion, while the waste products pass outwards through this same surface area. After the next division the cells are too numerous to continue as a compact mass which still allows each to have some access to the surface. To allow all cells to have contact with the nutrient fluid that bathes them, a hollow sphere is formed (Figure 6). A cleft appears in the middle of the cell group, and so all the cells retain a surface area through which they can be nourished. Soon one part of the sphere thickens and splits into two layers. From this disc all the tissues of the embryo develop.

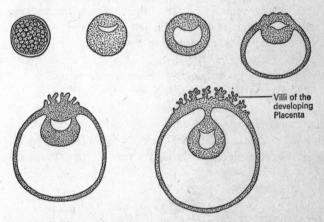

Villi of the developing Placenta

Figure 6. Development of a solid ball of cells which later forms a hollow sphere, to ensure each cell contact with the surrounding fluid.

While this cell-splitting is proceeding, the whole organism is being swept down the Fallopian tube towards the uterus, taking about 8–10 days. The uterine lining is prepared to receive the egg, and is thick and soft. Hormones from the ovary have caused this layer to grow rapidly, and much nutrient material is stored here. The ovum burrows into the uterine lining and so is surrounded by the mother's tissue and receives nourishment from the mother's blood. For the next 36 weeks the developing embryo is dependent for its oxygen and food on the mother, from whose blood these vital substances are obtained.

The Placenta

Once the embryo is embedded in the lining of the mother's uterus, all oxygen and food exchange must take place across the cells lining the sac in which it lies. Interchange occurs over the whole area and, to increase the surface available, finger-like processes grow into the mother's tissues (see Figure 6). These are called villi, and as well as providing a large exchange area, they anchor the embryo firmly in the mother's tissues.

The embryo grows rapidly, the sac coming to occupy the whole space available in the uterus. After 8–10 weeks, the villi retreat from over the larger part of the surface, and are concentrated over only a quarter of its area, which remains as a flat disc, attached firmly to the mother's tissues (Figure 7): this is the placenta, through which all communication

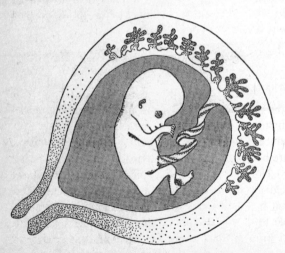

Figure 7. Uterus at about a 12-week pregnancy.

between the growing baby and mother is concentrated. It is often said that the placenta is the intra-uterine infant's lung, for it is the embryo's source of oxygen. By the same token it is the infant's kidney (excretion of waste products occurs here) and its liver (the placenta is used as a storage depot of foodstuffs). Any premature separation of the placenta from the mother's tissues may cause serious results for the infant. This is what occurs in a miscarriage and, more rarely, in certain forms of toxaemia of pregnancy (see Chapter 10).

All human tissue gets older with the passing of time. The placenta ages also; its life-span is required to be that of pregnancy only, but towards the end of that time degenerative changes occur, and the organ becomes less adequate. The shifting of oxygen to the baby and of waste products back to the mother's blood stream becomes less efficient. Obstetricians watch carefully for signs of placenta insufficiency especially when pregnancy continues after 40 weeks in a patient who is quite sure of her dates.

The Umbilical Cord

Joining the placenta to the embryo is a group of blood vessels. At first this consists of two arteries and two veins; later this is reduced to two arteries and one big vein. These blood vessels are bound together and carried in the umbilical cord (Figure 8). Notice how the vessels spiral in their course. They are packed inside the cord with a loose jelly which maintains them in position, rather as professional packers use newspaper to transport glass or china. The embryo's blood is carried from its body along the two umbilical arteries to the placenta. Here it is oxygenated and returned along the vein to be circulated around the growing body of the embryo.

The umbilical cord starts on the back of the placenta and carries the vessels to the navel of the baby. It is quite loose inside the embryonic sac to allow for, and to follow, the movements of the baby. In a tidal river no one would tie up a boat with a short rope, for the rising and falling of a closely tethered boat would soon cause it to sink. Similarly the cord must be long enough to let the infant move freely

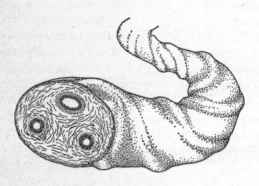

Fig. 8. Umbilical cord.

in its sac and still have an unrestricted blood supply. Most umbilical cords are about twenty inches long at full maturity, but the range of normal variation is considerable. Lengths from eight inches to five feet have been measured with perfectly normal babies.

After delivery, in the natural state, the blood vessels of the umbilical cord are tightly shut by spasm of the muscle of their walls. This cuts off the blood connexions between the baby and the placenta. Some animal species bite through the umbilical cord, but in human deliveries the obstetrician clamps or ties the cord tightly soon after the baby's birth. He then cuts the cord with a pair of scissors.

The Liquor

Figure 7 shows the developing embryo lying loose inside its sac. This allows for growth and movement. However, the infant is not hanging free like a lamp in a room. He is borne up by fluid as a fish is and so achieves a relatively weightless existence. Not only is he buffered by this fluid from mechanical shocks and alterations of the mother's position, but also temperature and noise variations are kept to a minimum.

The liquor that surrounds the embryo is derived partly from the infant's kidneys but mostly by perfusion from the mother's blood. It is constantly being produced and absorbed again, so that a steady state is reached, when the rates of production and reabsorption equal each other. Very occasionally this balance is disturbed. If too little fluid is made (oligamnios) the infant is pinched inside its sac, which fits it too well. The opposite situation, where there is excessive liquor, is called hydramnios: here there is far too much liquor, the baby floats around too freely and this may prevent the proper presentation of his head to the pelvis when labour starts.

Occasionally a doctor has to initiate labour earlier than nature intends. One of the best ways to do this is to let out some of the liquor. A simple and relatively pain-free procedure allows this to be done through the neck of the uterus with no more inconvenience than in a vaginal examination.

Development of the Organs

We have seen how the fertilized ovum implants itself and how it becomes a hollow sphere with a more specialized disc which is elaborated to form the future child (Figure 6). Development in the disc soon allows the laying-down of tissues and the specialization of these into individual organs. We shall now consider some of these.

The Brain and Nervous System

About sixteen days after conception, a column of cells running the length of the embryonic disc starts to thicken and sink beneath the surface, thus forming a trough. The edges of this come together and in a few days seal off the lips of the trench. A tube is formed, with the overlying skin sealed outside it. The sealing process begins in what will be the lower back region; it proceeds upwards towards the head and downwards towards the tail simultaneously.

At the head end, this new tube of potential nervous tissue expands in width and length. Since it is limited by the overlying skin, this fast growth can occur only by the kinking of the tube against the relatively fixed point of the head end of the embryo. Thus the head end of the nerve tube bends forwards and becomes convoluted, forming the complex pattern of the human brain.

Two mounds of tissue grow sideways from the central tube, and the very specialized upper brain is formed. It is here that all the higher functions are located. This complex organ has many cells and interconnecting pathways. During the months of early development, therefore, the surface area of the upper brain becomes greatly increased inside the skull by rapid growth, and by numerous folds which produce crevices in the surface. Figure 9 shows this increase in the complexity of the brain's surface at various stages of development.

While this growth is going on, every nerve cell in the brain and spinal cord is sending out nerve processes. These are strands of tissue connecting the cell with receptive sense organs, with other nerve cells or with muscles and organs. It

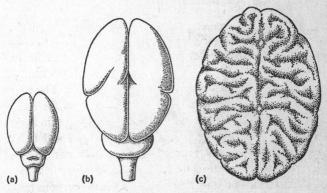

(a)   (b)   (c)

Figure 9. The brains of embryos at different stages of development. Notice the increasingly folded over surface of the cortex from (a) 12 weeks, (b) 24 weeks, and (c) 36 weeks of intra-uterine development.

is along these processes that impulses will travel carrying information to the central nervous system, and instigating motor activity in the muscles of the body. These processes are grouped together outside the spinal cord and brain, and form nerves that run to and from all parts of the body. As the limbs and organs develop, they carry these nervous processes with them, and are laying down the pathways for their future co-ordination in the body.

By about eight weeks of intra-uterine life the spinal cord is well formed and the brain is recognizable as such. The nerves have spread to the developing parts of the body, and all development from then on is of growth only. Certain nerves that carry particular impulses from the eye, ear and tongue develop directly from the brain but they are still of the basic pattern, being extensions of nerve tissue from the cells in the brain concerned with these particular sense organs.

The Sense Organs

A pair of hollow nerve processes grows forwards from the brain above the expanding nose. Approaching the overlying skin, the end of each process gets pushed in to form a cup (Figure 10) of two layers. The skin itself sinks into this cup,

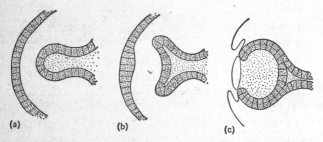

(a)   (b)   (c)

Figure 10. Development of the eye. Nerve process growing forward from brain (a), becoming cup-shaped (b). Overlying skin sinking in to meet cup and form conjunctiva covering eye ball (c).

forming the lens of the eye, and more skin-folds form the transparent front section of the eye and, subsequently, eye-lids.

A pair of similar dips and folds goes to form the ear on each side of the head. A tube of skin lining the throat grows upwards and outwards. This meets a pocket of skin from the side of the head forming the middle and outer ear and the eardrum between them. The inner ear, which provides hearing and balance sensations, is derived from an outgrowth of the nervous tissue from the brain base, which extends sideways to meet the two skin pouches. The outermost part of the ear, which is seen on the side of the head, comes from several skin projections that fuse together.

The Limbs

The embryo is at first sausage-shaped, but after twenty-eight days the brain grows rapidly, giving the embryo a recognizable head with eyes and ears. Before the fifth week of intra-uterine life, limb-buds are visible just behind the head and half-way along the body. They are tubes of skin filled with unspecialized tissue. This last forms the bones of the limb and the muscles that cover the bones. Joints appear at the future ankle, knee, hip, wrist, elbow and shoulder, and around them ligaments condense to strengthen the joints. At this stage the joints are simple gaps between the bones of the limbs, at which bending can occur, but soon a more complex arrangement is formed. The two bone surfaces in the joint grow in complementary shapes, one as a ball, the other a socket, thus making subsequent dislocation difficult. The bearing ends become coated with smooth cartilage, which facilitates movement at these joints.

The ends of the limbs flatten out like fans in which the small bones of the hands and feet differentiate. At first the fingers are joined together (see Figure 11) but later they separate, leaving only a small web of skin between them. Rarely, the end of the limb separates into six instead of five, and an accessory finger or toe is produced, which may be fused to another, or appear as a separate digit. This is not a serious abnormality and can be treated surgically if the parents wish. At the tips of the fingers and toes some of the cells of the skin thicken and sink deeper in, making a horny layer which grows forward – the nail.

As we saw previously, the nerves to the limbs all come as outgrowths from the spinal cord. These processes grow down the developing limbs and link up with sensory nerve endings in the skin, or to motor plates in the muscles. The hand, being our principal organ of fine discrimination, has a very rich nerve supply to its skin.

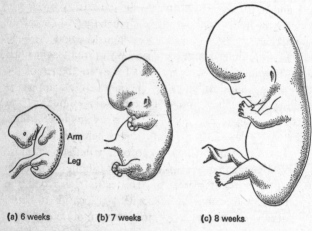

(a) 6 weeks   (b) 7 weeks   (c) 8 weeks

Figure 11. Development of the limbs.

Usually by the time the embryo is 5 weeks old the limbs are formed, with separate fingers and toes. At this stage the arms are usually at a further stage of development than the legs (see Plate 2). The nails are short and do not grow to reach the tips of the fingers until just before 40 weeks of intra-uterine life. Movements can be detected in the limbs by scientific methods at 8–10 weeks, but they are usually not noticed by the mother until later (16–20 weeks).

The Digestive Tract

The rapid growth at each end of the embryo causes the head and tail to overlap the ends of the embryonic disc (Figure 11), so that the linking yolk sac on the belly surface of the embryo becomes tucked in at the head and tail ends. The mass of the developing heart at one end and of the umbilical cord at the other soon forces this yolk surface to become contracted into a portion inside the developing embryo (the gut) and a pouch outside (the yolk sac). Unlike the bird embryo, the human does not obtain much nourishment from the yolk, and this sac soon shrinks. This leaves the part inside the embryo as a flattened tube running the length of the body. This gut tube grows more quickly than the rest of the body around it, and can find space for its growth only by twisting. The tube is suspended from the back of the

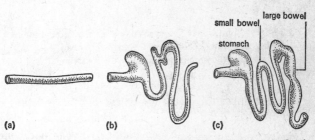

Figure 12. Development of the intestine. Rapid growth of a tube fixed at each end (a), results in convolutions (b). Dilatation occurs in some parts of the tube to form the different parts of the alimentary tract (c).

embryo's body, and as it twists loops occur. Some parts of the tube enlarge in diameter as well as in length. One of these local enlargements forms the stomach, another the large intestine.

41

In the head, the end of the gut tube comes in contact with a pit of skin that sinks in from the face, just below the nose (Figure 13a). The pit and tube join, so that the mouth cavity becomes continuous with the gut. The lips develop from bulges of skin that grow together (Figure 13b). The jaws come from the undifferentiated tissue under the skin, which hardens to form first cartilage and then bone (Figure 13c).

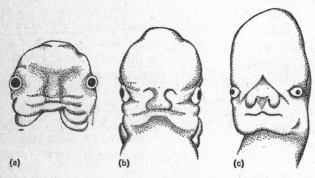

(a) (b) (c)

Figure 13. Development of the mouth. The eyes migrate round to the front of the face. The nose comes down from the forehead to fuse with a pair of tissue growths which form the upper lip. Occasionally the fusion is faulty and a hare lip results.

Over the upper rim of the lower jaw and the lower ridge of the upper jaw, little pits of skin sink into the developing cartilage. These produce in later life pegs of very hard bone – the teeth. From the floor of the mouth a ridge of muscle grows rapidly upwards and forwards, forming the tongue. This muscular organ is covered by expanding skin, from which taste buds develop.

From the sides of this common space a platform grows in, forming at the same time the floor of the nose and roof of the mouth. Occasionally a whole or a part of this platform is missing, so that the communication between nose and mouth persists, as a cleft palate. Modern surgical treatment can help to correct the disabilities of this deformity. If left untreated it would greatly interfere with both eating – food would go up into the nose – and speaking – air from the voice box would escape upwards, giving the voice a gross 'nasal' quality like an old-fashioned gramophone record.

The gullet or oesophagus passes from the mouth, through the chest to the stomach, where the tube has expanded (Figure 12) and acts as a storage area. The walls of the stomach are elastic and can be distended. This allows us to eat our food at intervals, taking in more than we immediately require. This food is kept and partly digested in the stomach, being released in small amounts to the rest of the digestive tract. When all the food has left the stomach, the sensation of hunger occurs and more food is taken. For most people in waking hours, the stomach requires replenishing about every four hours.

From the stomach, the 'gut' tube leads into the small intestine. This very convoluted tube is the main site of digestion and absorption of the food. It is about three feet long in the newborn infant. Anyone who has seen the inside of an animal at a butcher's shop must have been struck by the apparent disorder of the arrangement of the small intestine. In fact, it is suspended in an orderly fashion from the back wall of the body cavity by a sheet of connective tissue, through which all the blood vessels pass, carrying food-rich blood from the intestine to the rest of the body. The small intestine leads to the large intestine, a more capacious portion of the gut tube that runs around the edge of the body cavity. Here water is extracted from such food as remains undigested, so that the final waste products are both stored and dehydrated, before being evacuated from the body as faeces.

At the tail end of the body, the gut tube joints a pit in the tail skin to form the anus, in a fashion similar to that occurring at the mouth. This zone is surrounded by rings of muscle which act as a controlling mechanism, relaxing at will to allow faeces to pass out. Sometimes the anal pit of skin and the gut tube do not join. This results in an imperforate anus and obstruction to the bowel, though, if it is diagnosed promptly, surgery usually gives good results. Occasionally the muscle controlling the anus is defective. Then either lack of control allows incontinence, or spasm leading to retention of the faeces occurs, and here again corrective surgery may be helpful.

Blood and Blood Vessels

It has been shown earlier that, once a structure of many cells is developed, it is difficult for each cell to get its supply of nutrients or oxygen and to dispose of its waste products. Early in the embryo's growth, the cell mass becomes hollow, to allow all cells some contact with the bathing nutrient fluid. This method is practicable only with small numbers of cells. Soon embryonic development produces such a complex system of many layers that the surface method of nourishment is no longer possible. Hence an internal circulation of fluid is needed, to link every cell with the body's oxygen and food sources. This is the function of the blood stream; it is well adapted to the needs of a rapidly growing body with innumerable cells.

The blood contains red cells that carry oxygen to the tissues; these cells are floating in the plasma in which are dissolved foods diffused from the mother's blood. Four weeks after conception, groups of blood-forming cells gather in islands in all parts of the body. The cells at the edges of these islands join one another to form channels which proliferate in length, making arteries and veins. The central island cells produce red blood cells, while the fluid bathing the islands becomes plasma.

The primitive blood vessels (arteries and veins) grow rapidly into all developing tissues. Along the length of the embryo, a pair of big arteries is laid down in front of the spinal column. These are the main blood vessels, and blood circulates in them. As the embryo grows, a more efficient pumping mechanism is required to supply a faster and more continuous supply of oxygenated blood to the increased body bulk. In front of the gut tube in the chest region, the blood islands coalesce into a thick walled tube (Figure 14a).

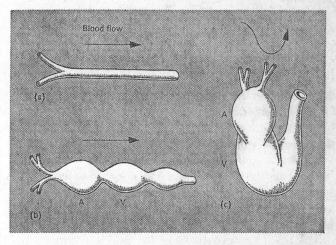

Figure 14. Development of the heart. The simple tube grows and because it is fixed at each end, it becomes more convoluted. The walls thicken and the action of the muscle in them pumps the blood around the body. A – Atrium chamber, V – Ventricle chamber.

This connects with the arteries and veins of the body and at five weeks starts a pumping action. Rapid growth of this tube, which is held firmly at each end, causes first, sacculation into compartments (Figure 14b) and later, bending of the tube itself (Figure 14c). The kinks thus produced develop into valvular folds so that the blood can flow only one way. Soon an incomplete partition grows down the middle of the organ and divides the two chambers seen in Figure 14 into the four chambers of the embryo's heart.

While the embryo is inside the mother's uterus, oxygenated blood comes from the placenta and not from the lungs, so the flow of the blood stream has to be modified for these different circumstances. Whereas after birth, blood from the right side of the heart is pumped through the lungs and returns fully oxygenated for dispersal by the left side of the heart to all the other tissues of the body, in the unborn child this route is useless, since the lungs are so far superfluous organs. These are by-passed by means of the incomplete partition between the two sides of the heart. The blood, which has received its oxygen as well as its foodstuffs from the placenta, enters the right side of the heart and passes directly through the hole in the partition to the left side. Usually, at birth, this hole closes when the lung circulation is established. Rarely, however, it stays open. This has the effect of continuing the intra-uterine by-pass mechanism, and so some of the baby's blood does not go to be reoxygenated in the lungs. The child is therefore at a lower oxygen level and is cyanosed – a blue baby. Advances in cardiac surgery in the last few years have made normal and healthy lives possible for children who, if they had been born thirty years ago, would either have died or been condemned to semi-invalidism.

The Lungs

From either side of the gut tube in the region of the chest two pouches form, spreading out into the chest cavity. These grow rapidly and convolute to form the lungs. Arteries and veins grow towards this tissue and branch many times to provide a rich blood supply in order that oxygenation of the blood can occur after birth. The front part of the gut tube in the upper chest and the neck separates into two; the back tube becoming the gullet, the front tube the windpipe.

In the uterus the embryo gets its oxygen from the placenta. The lungs are therefore not required, and are unexpanded, their blood supply being shunted past them. Though the lungs are not functioning organs, the embryo can make breathing movements, so that the chest wall moves rhythmically. The windpipe and the larger air tubes are filled with the liquid which is made in the lungs. At birth, the baby must empty the liquid from these tubes before he can breathe air. The squeezing of the chest during the baby's delivery down the birth canal of the mother helps in this; the attendant delivering the woman then sucks out as much fluid as he can with a special sucker as soon as the baby is born. This aspiration clears the mouth, nose and back of the baby's throat of a couple of teaspoonfuls of liquid.

Growth of the Embryo

Most of the changes described so far in this chapter take place in the first seven to nine weeks of pregnancy. It is during this time that most congenital abnormalities are laid down. Both interference with the natural processes of tubes dividing or joining, and the stunting of the growth of cells at vital partitions, can lead to defects in the body of the growing child. After this time, the embryo is complete, and further development is by growth only. Very few defects can start after these weeks. The vital importance of the mother's health in this early part of pregnancy must be stressed.

From conception to birth, the embryo grows at a very rapid rate, especially in the middle months of pregnancy. Table I. shows the length of the embryo and baby from

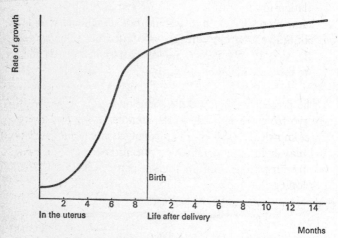

Table 1. Rate of growth of the embryo and newborn child. Observe the very fast rate of growth in mid-pregnancy.

conception through pregnancy and in the first year of life; in later pregnancy and early infancy the rate of growth is the same, but the mid-pregnancy rate is the fastest of any time. No limb or organ will ever grow as rapidly again. If this speed of growing were continued into later life, by 15 years the child would be 75 feet tall and weigh several tons.

Different parts of the body grow at different rates. The blood most rich in oxygen is conducted to the embryo's head end; the brain and head grow quickly, as is seen in Figure 11. The developing embryo looks big-headed, and at birth the head is still relatively large on the body. Some people retain a relatively large head into adult life, and if they go bald later, they look baby-like because of their head size.

The limbs of the embryo are of no use inside the uterus, and have a relatively poor blood supply. They look puny in relation to the rest of the body. Even after birth, for the first few months human babies do not use their limbs for weight bearing, and so growth is not fast. Once they start to toddle, the legs become stronger and grow longer in relation to the body.

The preceding pages have traced the development of an embryo from a single cell to the complex body of a baby. Exact knowledge of these stages is not essential, but the outline may help in understanding the precautions and procedures undertaken during pregnancy on behalf of the developing child.

3 | Knowledge of the Infant before Birth

Throughout pregnancy the unborn child is lying well protected by warm liquid inside the mother's uterus. This very protection makes investigation difficult; if we were theoretical biologists seeking to study a species, one of the last we would choose would be the human embryo. We have few means of getting at him, and so assessment of his progress is hard. Some of our methods of checking the infant in the uterus are time-honoured, some are new, and a few are still research projects. We really need a 'window in the uterus' so that we can learn more about what happens to the developing foetus. All the methods we discuss now help in building up a composite picture of the embryonic child's well-being.

Clinical Investigations

At intervals throughout pregnancy mothers attend ante-natal clinics and their health is checked by questioning and examination. It used to be thought that provided the mother was well, then the embryo inside her must also be thriving. The few infants of healthy mothers who were born mal-formed or ailing were thought to be manifestations of in-evitable acts of God, and it was considered impossible to avoid these afflictions. Nowadays we accept the blows of Fate less passively: and while there are still some tragedies which we cannot prevent, there are others which can be averted. Experience with Rhesus-affected babies and with those whose mothers had taken Thalidomide has amply emphasized this point. In both these groups the mothers were physically quite fit. Their unborn babies, however, were severely affected by the antibodies or the drug respectively crossing the placenta into the infant's circulation. Further, research procedures can detect the precarious nature of the infant's situation in the uterus while the mother is comparatively well in certain situations, as in the case of diabetes or mild degrees of hypertension (raised blood pressure).

Blood Pressure and Urine Testing

At each ante-natal clinic visit the mother's blood pressure is checked. Although wide variations can occur, once the patient is used to her surroundings the blood-pressure readings usually settle to a fairly constant level. This level is recorded, and the patient's urine is tested for the presence of protein or sugar. The presence of protein is an important diagnostic factor to be considered in conjunction with the blood-pressure recordings and will be discussed in the next paragraph. The presence of sugar in the urine may be an early sign of the forerunner of diabetes. Many women have some sugar in their urine during pregnancy, and this is not in itself serious: it is merely a reflection of the kidneys' different way of dealing with glucose metabolism in pregnancy. For a few who persistently show glucose in the urine, it is the early-warning sign of a pre-diabetic state, one that shows up only under the stress of pregnancy. These women may become diabetics later in life, and the progress of their unborn infants should be watched carefully in pregnancy and labour.

The blood pressure and presence of protein in the urine

are studied in conjunction with a third sign, that of the retention of fluid in the body. If water is stored in excess in the tissues, they become puffy. This shows in the ankles and lower legs. Most pregnant patients wear wedding rings and here puffiness of the fingers soon makes itself known. These three signs add up to toxaemia of pregnancy (now known as pre-eclampsia) and indicate that treatment is required. The relatively small rise in blood pressure is an example of a condition which rarely worries the mother; but the placenta and baby could suffer from the changes that such a toxaemia may produce. Hence the condition is treated vigorously at early stages. The treatment may include admission to hospital. This is usually resisted by the patient who feels quite normal, but the obstetrician is thinking of both mother and child, and it is wise to follow his advice for the baby's sake.

The Size of the Uterus

At each visit the size of the uterus is noted, and any relative increase from the last time is noted. Up until 20–24 weeks what the obstetrician is feeling is mainly an increase in the thickness of the muscle of the uterine wall and an increase of the liquor in the cavity. After 24 weeks, however, the parts of the baby can be detected, and from this time on the doctor is actually feeling the baby and his position in relation to the mother's pelvis (see Plate 3). It is useful to establish whether there is a regular increase in the size of the uterus, for in early pregnancy this is one of the signs of the infant's well-being which can be ascertained easily and without risk.

Occasionally the uterus is found to be bigger than is expected. In the first few months this discrepancy may be due to the fact that the pregnancy is further advanced than was thought. Many women have a little bleeding from the uterus in the early stages, and should this coincide with the date of an expected period it may be considered as such. In this case the pregnancy would be thought to have started four weeks later than it actually did. Careful questioning by the obstetrician often unveils this misunderstanding and explains the uterine size. Occasionally in early pregnancy the uterus may appear larger than expected because it was big at the start (after several previous pregnancies the uterus is often bulky) or because of the presence of fibroids. These are rounded masses of fibrous tissue which cause little harm but make the uterus bigger and so lead to confusion.

Should a gross enlargement of the uterus be noted only in the second half of pregnancy, one of the first diagnoses that come to mind is twins. From 24 to 30 weeks it is often possible to make a provisional diagnosis of twins; after this time the obstetrician can be more certain. One out of eighty pregnancies in Britain produces twins, of which about a sixth are identical twins from one egg.

Occasionally a uterus is excessively large because of an increase in the amount of fluid around the baby. Normally there is just enough fluid to insulate him from mechanical pressures and temperature variations; thus the quantity increases in proportion to the size of the baby as he gains weight. Sometimes the fluid production is excessive, and the infant bobs around like an apple at Hallowe'en. The position of the baby in the uterus is inconstant, for the uterine walls are stretched by the amount of fluid present and can no longer wrap and mould the baby into a head-down presentation to the pelvis. This situation occurs in fewer than 1 in 200 pregnancies and often the excess fluid is of no significance; but occasionally it warns the obstetrician of some defect in the gullet or intestine of the coming child. Each year many such abnormalities of the newborn are operated upon, and the results are good, provided the troubles are diagnosed early. This excess of fluid, therefore, can act as a warning sign in these rare cases.

At times the uterus appears smaller than expected. This too may be significant, but by far the commonest reason is that the patient is wrong in the dating of her pregnancy, which perhaps is not so far on as she thought. For example, should menstruation occur every forty-two days, instead of the supposed normal of twenty-eight, and ovulation is calculated to have occurred on the fourteenth day after the last period, the estimated length of pregnancy might be two weeks more than it really was. Not all women have a 28-day cycle, nor do they all ovulate on the fourteenth day. Moreover, some women produce smaller babies than average; in these cases the pregnant uterus will appear small for the estimated length of pregnancy, and it will be only after delivery that this can be known to be due to the size of the child. Further, patients who have raised blood pressure may produce smaller children. In rare cases in which the child dies during the pregnancy, the uterus may start to regress in size. If all movements have ceased for a week or so and the doctor cannot hear the baby's heart, this death may be confirmed by examination. Usually, a baby that dies is expelled from the mother's body fairly soon, but occasionally it is retained, with the subsequent sequelae of events mentioned above. However, these last are less common causes of a uterus being small; the most likely one is that the pregnancy is not as advanced as was thought.

Movements of the Infant

After the middle of pregnancy, the mother can feel the infant's limbs kicking and pushing as he churns around in the uterus. The time when the mother first becomes aware of these movements varies greatly. Some women are very sensitive to any intra-abdominal impressions; they notice, even in good health, the ripples of movement in their intestines and are sometimes agitated by them. Other women never notice their intestinal movements, and this second group do not feel a baby's kicking until later in pregnancy. Women who have had babies before know what the sensation of infantile restlessness is like and so recognize it sooner than women who are having their first babies. Generally speaking the latter group feel the baby kicking at about twenty to twenty-four weeks of pregnancy, while women with previous pregnancies notice movements up to four weeks before this.

At first the movements are faint, and it is difficult to be sure of their presence; but once established they get stronger. They vary greatly from one baby to another, some making their presence felt only once or twice a day, whereas others kick vigorously enough to wake their mothers from sleep. The presence of such movements is reassuring, but their absence does not prove that something is wrong, although it could be an indication that the infant is ailing. Alterations in movements are not a reliable guide to the progress of the infant.

Mary Tudor on two occasions, in 1554 and 1558, thought she was pregnant. She 'became large with child' and felt the baby's movements quite convincingly. On neither occasion was she really pregnant; she so earnestly desired a baby that her mind dictated to her body the signs of pregnancy, amongst which were the foetal movements. This 'pseudocyesis' or false pregnancy is not uncommon amongst those who greatly desire or greatly fear pregnancy, and it often continues to the stage where the patient is sure she is feeling movements while the obstetrician is sure that there is no baby present. The converse sometimes applies also. Women who have felt no movements for some weeks may be delivered of healthy, living children. Alteration in the baby's movements are probably not significant, but the obstetrician should be consulted if they persist for some time.

The Heart Beat

In the last three months of pregnancy the baby's heart can be heard by the obstetrician. It is much faster than the adult pulse, going at 130–50 beats a minute (compared with the adult's 70–90 beats). It sounds like a big watch through a pillow, being slightly muffled by the layers of fluid, uterus and mother's abdominal wall. Many doctors listen to the infant's heart with a special wide-mouthed tube (see Plate 4), but it can equally well be heard with an ordinary stethoscope. It is obviously best heard through the baby's chest or upper back, and so it is useful if the baby's position has been determined accurately beforehand. This cannot be done until the later weeks of pregnancy. Further, a large amount of fluid around the baby, thickness of the uterus and a substantial amount of fat on the mother's abdominal wall all make the sounds more difficult to hear.

The rate of the heart beat is a reliable guide to the unborn baby's state since it can be checked easily and quickly. At the ante-natal clinic it is listened to at each visit; in labour the baby's heart is frequently sounded, and at this time is probably the best clinical guide to his well-being. Throughout labour, uterine contractions occur regularly, and these may cause a temporary diminution of the blood supply to the placenta and so to the child. This is reflected in a temporary, mild alteration of the heart rate. If, however, the infant is getting short of oxygen over a longer period, a greater alteration occurs. This is sometimes a warning sign to the obstetrician to take certain steps, which are discussed later.

Lack of oxygen is not the only cause of alteration in the foetal heart rate. The mother may have a mild infection (such as influenza) and so have a temperature. As a part of the body's natural reaction to infection, both her own and her baby's heart rate will go up. Similarly certain medicines given to the mother in labour can cause an alteration in the baby's heart rate which is quite normal. Conversely, as the infant's head is passing through the bony passages of the pelvis, it is compressed; this too is a normal and natural event, but it causes a temporary slowing of the heart rate. All these extra factors are taken into consideration by the obstetrician when assessing a baby's progress throughout labour.

X-Rays and Sound-Wave Investigations

X-rays are similar to light waves except that they are much more penetrating. Like light waves, they can pass through certain substances but are stopped, partly or wholly, by other materials. Photographically sensitive films can pick up X-rays after they have been beamed through the body. Just as light waves passing through glass, thin paper, and parchment give a graded effect on a film, so X-rays penetrating muscle, cartilage or bone give rise to a variated photographic picture. Since X-rays were discovered by Röentgen in 1895, they have been used to show up parts of the body inaccessible to the eye, such as the contents of the abdomen of a pregnant woman. From about eighteen to twenty weeks onwards the baby's developing bones contain enough calcium to show on an X-ray film. As he grows in size the X-rays become clearer (see Plate 5).

Used carefully, X-rays can be of immense use to the obstetrician. The presence of twins, if suspected, can be confirmed (see Plate 6). The position of the infant in the uterus can be checked. The size of the baby may be estimated, and, from calculations on the bone growth, a rough idea of his maturity may help the doctor if there is doubt about the duration of pregnancy. The mother's pelvis can be measured with a greater degree of accuracy than with an examining finger. Occasionally some malformations of the infant's skeleton can be discovered. Several finer details of the exact way the baby is liable to proceed in labour can be evaluated, and may be of help to the obstetrician conducting the case.

With all these advantages, it might seem surprising that most women are not X-rayed during their pregnancy when one or another of the various factors mentioned is relevant. Certainly X-rays opened up a new dimension in ante-natal diagnosis, and just after the Second World War they were used widely, even indiscriminately, to help diagnosis. However, in the 1950s doctors began to realize that irradiation might have undesirable side effects. Sometimes the marrow cells of the developing baby were stimulated so that abnormalities of the blood occurred after birth. Occasionally, if the X-ray was taken while the embryo was at a critical early stage of development, before twelve weeks maturity, organs might be stunted and so an abnormality could result.

As a result of the fears of these possibilities, there was a wave of reaction against X-rays in Britain, and they came to be used much less frequently. These fears represented an over-exaggeration of the true position. The two risks mentioned are both much less serious than the risk to the baby of an unsuspected twin being present or of a delivery attempted through a pelvis not suitable for him. Hence common sense is now causing doctors to swing back to the idea that ante-natal X-rays can be taken when they are indicated. Even so we now use them far less than fifteen years ago. When, then, an obstetrician orders such an investigation, he has already considered the risks and calculated that they are not serious enough to outweigh the more immediate consideration of producing a live and healthy baby.

Recently sound waves have been used to give composite pictures of the child in the uterus. This method (Sonar) is fresh from the research field, and only a few centres in Britain are equipped for such an investigation. The sound waves are 'bounced off' hard objects, such as the baby's bones, and their reflections are photographed. Thus a picture of the infant can be built up. The whole principle is complex but works in the same way as Asdic does in detecting submarines under water. Sound waves are free of the potential hazards that exist with irradiation, and good images can be obtained, especially of the child's skull (see Plate 7). The pictures require expert interpretation, but those who work much with these methods pronounce them capable of giving as good results as conventional X-rays, and in some situations better.

Most methods of investigation discussed so far are in clinical use and, with the exception of the last, can be applied at any ante-natal centre in Britain. They are time-honoured, and interpretation of their results is, in the hands of experienced obstetricians, a major factor in assessing the unborn infant's progress and welfare. However, these methods of observing the infant in his environment are being expanded by ancillary tests. Some of these are almost routine in larger centres that have research laboratories;

others are at a more preliminary stage and their usefulness is still being assessed.

The Electrical Activity of the Foetal Heart

Every time a muscle contracts, it gives off a small electrical discharge. This electrical activity can be picked up on the skin, amplified and recorded. An adult's heart muscle activity has been measurable for years by electrocardiography. When doctors wish to know more about a patient's heart actions, they can record the electrical output by this simple and quick means. It has been much harder to examine the unborn baby's heart electrically, for two reasons. Firstly, it has a much smaller electrical output, about a twentieth of that of an adult. Secondly, it is harder to pick up the feeble impulse emanating from so deep inside the mother's muscles. The uterus and maternal abdominal wall have their own electrical activity. Thus much complex electronic analytical equipment is required to filter out the foetal heart beats from the background electrical signals. However with such apparatus the rate and rhythm of the unborn infant's heart can be monitored effectively (Figure 15).

Many of the difficulties that the complex electronic signal causes are due to the indirect methods of recording through the mother's abdominal wall. Once the membranes around the infant have ruptured and the cervix of the uterus starts to dilate, electrodes can be attached directly to the baby's scalp. Now the investigator obtains a much purer recording of the baby's own heart action without the extraneous electrical activity of the mother's muscles. These direct records are easier to interpret, but, because of the way the infant is placed in the uterus, they can best be obtained when the mother is close to, or in, labour; hence they are of use only at the very end of pregnancy. This is not a great disadvantage, for it is mostly at this time that the obstetrician requires an accurate and speedy guide to the foetal state. Because the electrodes are placed directly on foetal skin, a cleaner electrical tracing is obtained.

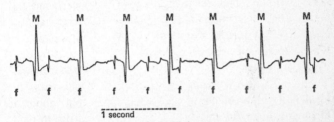

Figure 15. An electrical reading of the unborn baby's heart. The peaks marked M are recorded from the mother's heart. They are at a much slower rate than those marked f which are recorded from the baby's heart.

There is still more research to be done in this field. Electrocardiograph recordings of the adult heart can be examined in detail to determine the state of oxygenation of the heart's cells. The shape of the trace and its relation to the amount of electrical output can be closely correlated with the heart cells' biochemical state. Up to now, the foetal electrocardiograph has been too crude to allow analysis of its wave form. It has been of use as a rate meter only, and so only quantitative results could be expected from it. The newer, direct records will allow a more qualitative analysis, and rapid assessment of the unborn child's heart's electrical, and so biochemical, state will be possible.

Electrically Amplifying the Baby's Heart Sounds

As mentioned before, from twenty-eight weeks the baby's heart can be heard by the obstetrician. If, instead of a stethoscope, a microphone is put over the loudest source of the foetal heart sounds, these can be picked up and amplified for transmission over a loudspeaker, which can be positioned at any distance from the patient. One advantage of phonocardiography is that the microphone can be applied and comfortably held in place by an elastic belt, allowing the patient to sleep without disturbance of doctors or midwives examining her for continuous checking. A disadvantage is that when the child moves in the uterus the microphone may no longer be over the point where heart sounds can best be heard, and so it has to be reapplied. Probably, phonocardiography is a useful subject for research but at present has few advantages over a good midwife listening through a conventional stethoscope.

Hormone Measurement

In Chapter 2, the function of the placenta as a transporter of oxygen was discussed. However, this organ has many other functions to play in pregnancy. Oestrogen (really a complex of several related hormones) controls the growth and function of the pregnant uterus and may affect the mother's milk production. The other group of hormones, the progesterones, is important in the protection of the foetus. The uterus, like any hollow muscular organ, has a natural tendency to contract, and progesterone reduces the muscle tone so making contraction less likely. The production of these hormones by the placenta is essential to the continuation of pregnancy. It is possible to measure the amounts in the blood of the mother, or in her urine after the hormones have been excreted by the kidneys, but the techniques for these estimates are difficult and practised in only a few hospitals.

As pregnancy progresses, the hormone concentration rises (Table 2). This increase is roughly proportional to the increase in the bulk of the functioning placenta, and is sometimes used as a guide to the efficiency of the organ in

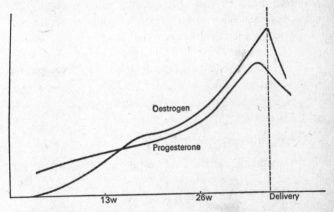

*Table 2.*Increase in hormone levels as pregnancy advances. The increase is roughly proportional to the bulk of the functioning placenta.

other directions, for instance in the transport of oxygen to the foetus. It has not been proved that there is a direct relationship between these different functions of the placenta in the way that this reasoning implies; however, if an unborn baby seems not to be thriving and if the necessary equipment is available, it may be worth estimating the oestrogen output of the placenta. If this shows a falling off, it is reasonable to assume that the placenta may also be failing to oxygenate the foetal blood, and this might indicate the necessity to induce labour immediately, in order to improve the baby's chance of survival.

At present these hormone assays are not advanced enough for routine use. They can be performed only in special centres; they are difficult and time-consuming to perform and require specially skilled staff to get accurate results; further, the details of their interpretation have not been worked out fully. To do one or two estimations on any mother at the latter end of pregnancy is not enough. The hormone assays have to be performed at intervals during that patient's pregnancy in order that the change in the patient's hormone level can be appreciated. At present, much research time is taken up by the further development of these tests.

Direct Examination of the Baby's Blood

All the methods, clinical and research, mentioned so far produce indirect estimations of the progress of the infant or his placenta. Up to now it has been difficult to reach the unborn baby directly, but in the last few years an ingenious method has been developed in West Berlin by a German obstetrician, Ehrich Saling. The idea was introduced to Britain by Professor Peter Huntingford, and much work has been done by Dr Richard Beard at Queen Charlotte's Hospital, developing and refining the method. Now it is being taken up in several maternity hospitals, but it requires expert laboratory techniques and so is not yet available in every obstetric unit. Shortly before labour most babies lie with the head just over the cervix. A narrow tube is passed through the cervix and a small drop of blood is drawn from the baby's scalp while it is still inside the uterus. The tube in the vagina is not painful to the mother and the small pin-prick in the infant's scalp is no more than that used to give an intramuscular injection. Along a second specially pre-pared tube, a bead of the baby's blood can be drawn and then taken away for analysis. This allows accurate and im-mediate assessment of the baby's state of oxygenation. So valuable is this method that one large maternity hospital in London is applying it to all mothers in labour whose babies may be in difficulty. Obviously it can be used only when the cervix is a little open. This, in the first pregnancy, usually means after labour has started, but the cervix of a woman who has had a baby before is often gaping enough in the last week of pregnancy to allow the test to be performed then.

The direct measurement of the baby's state of oxygena-tion is a most important investigation and may soon move from the research laboratory to use in many more obstet-ric hospitals. It is the most direct of all the 'windows on the uterus' that we have, for now we are recording directly from the unborn infant's tissues. Before this test was evolved, we were measuring the effects of foetal events on various extra-uterine and intra-uterine organs. The re-sponses of these organs themselves added another variable and so made the tests less accurate. Intra-uterine foetal blood sampling is opening up new avenues for exploration of life on the far side of the placenta.

All the investigations discussed in this chapter aim to give information about the child inside the uterus. Finally, how-ever, it is your obstetrician who has to correlate the facts he discovers with his experience of past situations, and on this he acts. When he is caring for a patient ante-natally, it is always of the double mother/child relationship that he is thinking and for the welfare of both that he recommends treatment.

2 | Congenital Anomalies

4 | The Extent of the Problem

In the collective memory of the community, it is the mis-adventures which are most easily recalled: unpleasant events, it seems, imprint themselves most indelibly on the mind. It is difficult, therefore, to make an exact appraisal of the frequency of abnormalities in babies; the abnormal attracts more attention than the normal, and its incidence is thus grossly exaggerated. The hundreds of normal babies are crowded out of the memory by the one that is not perfect.

In Great Britain all doctors are statutorily obliged to certify death. No burial or cremation can occur without such a certificate, and so it is probable that a fairly accurate estimate of the death rate in the country can be obtained from the Registrar General's figures. Since the age of the deceased appears on such a certificate, the neonatal death rate (that is, of those who die within a month of birth) can easily be calculated. Similarly certificates must be given for all babies who are born dead. No such regulations existed for notifying congenital abnormalities until a few years ago, when some local authorities (the late London County Council among them) started a system of registering such affected children. There is a difficulty here, however, which does not arise in the case of the registration of death, and which has to do with the problem of diagnosis. Death is a finite occurrence that any doctor can detect and certify, but a minor abnormality of the foot or nervous system of a newborn child could be missed or only just suspected. Hence certification of the abnormality would be delayed, or might even never take place at all.

Several scientific surveys have been performed to try to assess the incidence of abnormal babies. The Liverpool region has been fortunate for years in having Professor R. W. Smithells working on this problem, and he estimates that he is informed of at least ninety per cent of the abnormalities in this large region. Several smaller surveys confirm this figure.

From the Registrar General's statistics, we can tell that 20 out of every 1,000 mature babies are liable to be born dead, while a further 15 may die in the first week of life. This is a time of maximum risk: an individual stands a greater chance of dying at this period than at any time in the next forty years. The reasons for these deaths will be discussed in the next few chapters, but the principal three are congenital abnormalities, interference with the oxygen supply of the baby while in the uterus and breathing difficulties encountered by the baby in the first minutes or hours of life.

Congenital abnormalities in the human race are very rare, but, as we have seen, the exact figures are hard to come by. Some defects may be obvious at birth to both medical and lay onlookers. These will be reported, and some figures will be obtained. However, there are some anomalies which are internal, and a few of those do not make themselves manifest until later childhood or even adult life. Certain heart irregularities in young men were not picked up until the sufferers had a medical examination before doing National Service. Insurance medical assessors can give numberless examples of cases in which congenital defects were uncovered only when the potential policy holder was examined at the age of twenty-five or thirty. Recently a doctor in America followed five thousand women through pregnancy. He and a team of paediatricians carefully examined each infant at birth, then at one month, a year and five years later. Seeking carefully for abnormalities, he found that about half of the total number discovered were found within the first month of life. It must be stressed that the other fifty per cent included many non-important variations of the normal which would probably not have affected a child's life. It is the more serious anomalies which are usually identified very soon after birth.

In Britain probably only twenty live babies in each thousand have any abnormality, and this may range from serious heart disease to an extra skin tag in front of the external ear. These figures represent the obvious abnormalities which are detected in the first few days of life. Thus two per cent of the infants born in Britain show some degree of malformation. This is a background figure that gives no information about the relation between such abnormalities and events that may have happened to mothers during pregnancy; this aspect will be discussed in the next chapter. Despite the figures given in this paragraph, probably only about another fifteen infants of every thousand live births will show any further stigmata of congenital malformation later in life. Thus a careful examination of the newborn baby will probably find any serious malformations and can give the parents real reassurance.

So far in this chapter only mature infants have been discussed. It is conventional to consider any infants who have grown in the uterus to twenty-eight weeks to be potentially viable. If an infant is expelled before this stage the patient is considered to have aborted or miscarried. Two of the principal causes of deaths which occur at this earlier time in pregnancy are congenital abnormalities and intra-uterine deprivation of oxygen. Again, exact figures of the number of pregnancies that miscarry are impossible to obtain. Some women may miscarry so early that they were not aware of being pregnant at all. Others may have reasons for wishing to conceal their pregnancy (and its termination) and so may not seek medical aid. However, informed estimates are that about a fifth of all pregnancies in Britain miscarry. This means that they terminate before the infant is large enough to live outside the uterus. The majority of such abortions come in the eighth to twelfth week of pregnancy, and, although some may be criminally induced, at least half of them occur spontaneously. Careful medical examination of such abortions shows that many of the embryos which abort spontaneously are malformed and not fit to stand even the protected life they led in the uterus. They would have been even less adapted to the hurly-burly of extra-uterine life, and this seems Nature's way of preventing too many abnormal children being born. Natural selection ensures that abnormal members of a species are discouraged from reproducing themselves; spontaneous abortion may be an extreme example of this natural rule.

These two examples, abnormalities found later in life and abortions, show how difficult it is to give exact statistics about the numbers of children affected in the uterus by any given factor. In the following chapters, the various influences that may jeopardize the safety of the unborn child will be discussed in some detail, and, against the background of what has been said before, the risks involved in individual cases will be assessed.

5 | Searching for Causes

Every woman hopes that her baby will be born without blemish. As was said earlier, the fear of an abnormal child often weighs more heavily on the mind than the fear of a dead baby. In Britain, forty-nine out of fifty babies born alive are normal. The exceptional baby does have some defect that can be traced back to a fault in development. Chapter 2 showed the complex mechanisms involved in the growth of a fully mature infant from a single fertilized cell. It is not hard to imagine that any interference occurring at a critical stage in cell division could alter the whole pattern of further growth, division or fusion of the tissues. A fault built into any system is perpetuated as that system grows and is carried to all the parts that evolve from the defective area. If, at the stage of heart development, damage should occur to one of the cells of the septum dividing the heart into two sides, a gap might be left in that partition so that a permanent hole would exist. This would lead to some degree of mixing of the oxygenated and unoxygenated blood and so a cyanosed or blue baby might be born. Similarly, a flaw could occur to a few cells concerned with the channels containing the fluid that fills and bathes the nervous system. If the circulation of this fluid is dammed back, it collects inside the skull and causes it to become abnormally large. This condition is hydrocephalus, or water on the brain, and unless the trapped fluid is released the child's nervous system may be impaired.

Sometimes errors in development stem from an inbred

fault inherited from one or other of the parents. In others some factor from outside has altered the equilibrium of the infant's environment. Most of the time we cannot recognize that factor. The next chapters contain accounts of a few of the agents known to be responsible for causing malformations, and an account of how we can learn more about the babies affected by them, for thorough knowledge might enable us to avoid the damaging external factors.

The writer once delivered a woman who had a baby with an abnormal heart. The baby died in five days, and an examination showed gross alterations in the heart's structure that would not have been compatible with his survival in the outside world. The patient had a normal child of two years at home and wondered why this time she had been visited with an abnormal pregnancy. Going back over her medical story, we found no occurrence of any congenital abnormalities in her family or in that of her husband. In addition to this she had already been delivered of one normal baby, so that no genetic factors need have been involved. The patient attributed the catastrophe to an anti-sickness drug that she had taken during the first three months of pregnancy. But as well as this drug, she had consumed a lot of aspirin in the same three months; and she had also taken iron tablets (prescribed by the ante-natal clinic) and vitamin tablets (bought from the local chemist). Several nights, being unable to sleep, she had helped herself to some of her husband's sleeping tablets. Christmas came when she was about seven weeks pregnant; she went to at least three parties, where she drank some alcohol though not enough to become inebriated. When nine weeks pregnant, she caught flu and had a temperature of 102–3° F.; this was treated with more aspirin and rest in bed. At about six weeks of pregnancy she had had a spotting of blood from the vagina, which lasted two days; she thought she was threatening to miscarry and so rested in bed for a couple of days. Further, she remembered, on looking back, that some two to three weeks after conception she had burnt her wrist badly on a saucepan in her kitchen. This caused a lot of pain and subsequent blistering. Such an incident would certainly cause the release of extra adrenalin from the suprarenal glands into her general circulation.

Here is a patient who presents us with ten factors each of which has at some time been considered as a possible cause of abnormalities; yet they have occurred in the pregnancies of millions of women who have subsequently produced perfectly normal babies. They are all dramatic things that the patient could, when it was necessary, recall. Did any of them cause her baby to have an abnormal heart? There were so many possibilities that neither she nor her medical advisers could sort out the wheat from the chaff. To identify the relevant alteration in the patient's life, which may have been very trivial, is impossible, since we have no certain means of screening out the irrelevant. To overcome the difficulties caused by forgetfulness and by the natural propensity to lay the blame on irrelevant events, other methods of investigation must be sought. At present there are three ways in which congenital abnormalities are investigated.

Methods of Investigation

In medical research, the investigator can either work with the incidents that occur in a random fashion or try to control the external factors to limit the number of variables. The first mode of inquiry is the only one possible with

75

human patients; the second is hard to apply to humans and we have to rely on animal work for such studies.

In the epidemiological field, in order to find the cause of human abnormalities a full survey of the environment must be made. This may be done by making inquiries after the abnormality is diagnosed (retrospective surveying) or by following a group of patients through their pregnancy and then comparing the data of the whole group with those of patients where malformations are found (prospective surveying).

Retrospective Surveys

Formerly the only method of correlating congenital abnormalities with environmental events was by inquiring back about the pregnancy and past history of the mothers who had produced abnormal babies. Unfortunately, maternal memories, and even the attending doctors' memories, are remarkably unsure some months after the event. When trying to puzzle out the reasons for inexplicable events, the human brain rationalizes and is notoriously unreliable as a source of objective information. A great help in the surveys of abnormalities has been good medical records with details of illnesses and of the drugs prescribed. However, the busy doctor on his round, or in his crowded surgery, usually writes brief notes and the relevant details may well not be recorded.

In March 1958 a national retrospective survey was mounted in Great Britain: the Perinatal Mortality Survey. As far as possible all deliveries in one week of March that year were most carefully scrutinized. The 17,205 deliveries examined were estimated to represent about ninety-eight per cent of the total number of births that week. In all these cases a comprehensive questionnaire was filled in, covering details of the mother's pregnancy and labour, social and family background and past health, and the early days of the infant's life. These facts were recorded in great detail, and the whole survey was then analysed. As can be imagined, even with computer help this was a massive undertaking. It has been estimated that, if all the information received had been coded, a vast number of permutations could have been expressed, probably in the range of 10 to the 480th power. A lot of the correlations would not be useful, however, and so much selection had to be made to sift out the meaningful facts. In this way a great deal of valuable information was obtained for use by obstetricians.

In 1960 the effects of Thalidomide on the unborn child were noted. This drug is discussed in the next chapter, but it is interesting to note here that its harmful nature was suspected from a retrospective inquiry.

These are two examples of useful retrospective surveys. Their effectiveness, however, was due to the all-embracing nature of the inquiry in the first instance and the rather unusual nature of the abnormalities caused by Thalidomide in the second. Not all retrospective surveys either investigate the environment so thoroughly or deal with so specific a situation. They are usually more limited in nature and depend too much on vague and naturally biased data. They are probably of less general use than planned prospective work.

Prospective Surveys

This type of investigation aims to follow a group of pregnant women from the earliest days of pregnancy. Potentially relevant events are recorded as they happen and are later correlated with any abnormalities found after delivery.

Prospective surveys thus have the advantage of working with unusually accurate information.

There are, however, two grave difficulties. The first is that at the start one does not know which facts are likely to be relevant. Much data must therefore be included which may be unnecessary when the final analysis is made. It was said at a recent medical conference on the subject that so many variables might be involved that only one person could keep a close enough watch – the patient. She would have to be asked to keep a detailed diary of early pregnancy, recording not only details of the medicines and drugs she took, but also of all the food she ate, what she did every minute of the day, the state of the weather, and even which television programmes she watched. This is obviously impossible, but it gives an idea of the amount of detail required for a general survey. In consequence, prospective surveys often concentrate on one specific factor. An investigation of this sort was recently conducted by Professor Smithells in Liverpool, in relation to a commonly used anti-vomiting treatment (details of this work appear in Chapter 8). Single-factor surveys are much easier to plan than multifactorial ones, and most workers now confine themselves to this sort of prospective inquiry.

The second difficulty is that a large number of mothers must be included at the beginning of a prospective inquiry into causes of congenital abnormalities. No one can tell which women will have affected children. Further, a certain number of women will move away from the area, or else default from the clinics and so be lost from the inquiry. Hence a large group must be started in order to get a reasonable return at the end of the survey.

Animal Work

In an effort to estimate the effects of external events on the unborn child, animal experiments are useful. No human lives are endangered, and the work can be pushed to the point of death in order to gain knowledge that may save children. Apart from the anti-vivisection point of view, there are, however, scientific objections to this type of work. All species react differently to potentially harmful agents. Given the same external stimulus at comparable stages of pregnancy, different animal species can produce different degrees of the same malformation or an entirely different malformation, or even no malformation at all. Two examples illustrate this. High doses of cortisone given to pregnant mice and rabbits at a certain time cause cleft palates in the offspring, but this effect is not obtained in rats. Even after Thalidomide was known to be a danger to the unborn human baby, it was very difficult to find another species that had the same susceptibility. All the commoner laboratory animals were tested, but not until the New Zealand white rabbit was used was the harmful effects of Thalidomide reproduced. Hence to get as accurate a result as possible, many different species at different stages of pregnancy must be tested with various intensities of a suspected agent. It is false to assume a direct correlation between experiments on animals and on humans, but extrapolation of one to the other may give some clues.

This work, even if the accuracy is acceptable, is time-consuming. Sometimes testing a drug at a very early stage of animal embryo development may be helpful. A Cambridge research worker, Dr Ludwig Mann, has perfected a technique of recovering from a pregnant rabbit the immature bundle of cells developed six and a half days after fertilization. During this time the rabbit may have been given various drugs or subjected to X-rays or alterations of temperature. After removal, the embryos are examined microscopically, and alterations in their structure can be seen. Not only drugs but vitamins and hormones are being checked by this method.

All these methods of investigation are leading us to a fuller knowledge of the causes of congenital abnormalities. Some of these we can prevent, and the chapters that follow describe how research along the outlines above has helped to reduce the production of abnormal children.

6 | Genetic Causes

The recognized causes of development errors may be grouped into inborn faults and outside factors. The first are inherited from the parents and are called genetic, for they are passed in the genes. We know least about these inborn errors, and a discussion of them is of necessity limited. The second group are environmental and will be dealt with in Chapter 7.

We all derive our physical characteristics from our parents; possibly even the biochemical bases of thought processes are inherited. Such transmitted factors are carried in the genes from the father and mother. Genes are microscopic tissues strung together like a bead necklace to make a chromosome (see Plate 8), twenty-three of which are contained in each sperm and ovum. Every chromosome is made up of hundreds of genes, each of which in turn carries the many characteristics of the future child. When the sperm and ovum fuse, the two chains of chromosomes come to lie alongside each other, fitting together like two strings of pearls twisted together. From here on, at every cell division the chromosomes divide inside the cell's nucleus; thus every cell in the body carries the baby's potential characteristics handed down from the parents.

After almost all these divisions, the two cells so produced have exactly the same genetical pattern as the parent cell, but occasionally variations in the division of the chromosomal groups occur so that unbalanced numbers of genes go to each of the cells. These are known as mutations, and represent alterations in the cellular genetic make-up; they occur in humans about three times in every ten thousand cell divisions. Most of these improper chromosome cleavages are so harmful to life that the cell is killed. Should the change be less lethal, however, the cell may live in a modified form. Most of the millions of cells in the body are not essential individually, but act in groups. Mutation in the nuclei of these cells usually causes no harm: but if the mutation occurs in a cell which forms an essential keystone in one of the body's vital systems, and if this takes place at the precise moment of foetal development when that system is being laid down, then a congenital malformation may follow.

Such abnormalities occur only at critical phases of development; some may be so severe that the baby dies in the uterus soon after the conception (an abortion), later in pregnancy (a stillbirth) or soon after delivery (a neonatal death). As in these instances the individual dies long before he can reproduce, the abnormalities will not be handed on to the next generation and so are self-limiting. A lesser degree of cellular damage may not lead to death; in such cases babies could grow to adulthood and possibly reproduce the defect in their offspring.

Abnormalities may occur in children of both sexes (for example, hare lip), or of one sex only (for example, haemophilia, which is confined to male children). The trouble may be obvious at birth, like cleft palate, or in early life, like congenital dislocation of the hip, or it may not become apparent until much later in life, like multiple cysts of the kidneys, or some mild forms of congenital heart disease.

Advances in medical treatment may now, paradoxically, be increasing the number of genetically caused congenital diseases. Until a few years ago, children with certain forms of heart disease seldom lived long enough to reproduce. The few who did were too ill to be socially acceptable as partners in marriage. Hence the malformation was a genetic cul-de-sac in evolutionary progress. Heart surgeons are now correcting many of these defects, restoring the individual to full health and active life. They are not, however, correcting the genetic background of the children, but are making it possible for them to survive, to marry and have children; so it is possible that the number of affected children will now rise.

It is these inherited abnormalities that we know least about and have least power to prevent. Humans meet, fall in love, marry and breed in a haphazard fashion, and to try to control human mating would be considered an intolerable attack on the freedom of the individual. Generally it is for medicine to help the offspring of genetically inadvisable marriages rather than to dictate that such marriages shall not occur. Many people do not realize that the Church has been active in this field for centuries. At the end of the Anglican Prayer Book, after the Thirty-nine Articles and the Ratification Charter, appears a page that has mystified many: 'A Table of Kindred and Affinity wherein whosoever are related are forbidden by the Church of England to marry together'; similar injunctions exist in the other Christian and in most of the non-Christian sects. The English table goes on to forbid marriage to twenty-five of one's kin. Figure 16 shows how these represent all the women around a man who might be carrying the same family genetic diseases. Many of these congenital defects will appear only if both parents' genes are affected. So the Church deemed it wise to keep such people apart, thereby reducing the risk of producing abnormal infants. There have been families powerful enough to circumvent the Church's edicts on this. The Spanish royal family continually inter-married with their own cousins, and in consequence haemophilia appeared in most of the male children. The

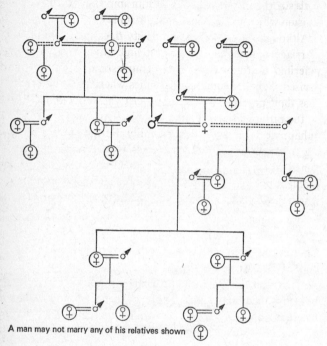

A man may not marry any of his relatives shown ♀

Figure 16. 'A man may not marry his . . .'
Representation of how one male and his female relations might all carry the same family diseases.

Hapsburgs of Austria inbred similarly, and their familiar jaw and lip appeared from generation to generation. Some primitive societies place an absolute ban on marriage to anyone with a congenital deformity, hoping to reduce abnormalities. Certain totalitarian states in Europe tried a similar manoeuvre in the 1930s. Whether the incidence of abnormality was significantly reduced or not, neither group succeeded in abolishing genetic malformations, for no ban of this sort can prevent the random improper chromosome division which causes them in the first place.

Although an emancipated society does not prohibit the marriage of couples who are at high risk of reproducing inherited malformations, these couples can be guided and advised. Some hospitals have clinics where parents can discuss their problems with a geneticist; he can counsel them on the probabilities of future trouble. This course may save unhappiness and tragedy in a family. Further ways of helping to prevent the birth of infants with genetically determined anomalies are discussed in Chapter 9. This is a problem both of the individual couple and of the society in which they live. It is for each to help the other to solve it.

7 | Environmental Causes

Many outside influences are known to be harmful to the developing infant, and in the next few years we shall undoubtedly find others. It is possible that the nature of the agent is not the only important factor in producing any abnormality. The timing of its noxious influence at a critical stage in the development or growth of the embryo may be as significant as the agent itself.

Early in development, at the time when the embryo is just embedding, a harmful stimulus often causes an all-or-nothing response, the embryo being either unharmed or else killed. The tissues are undifferentiated, and no organs have started to form. Hence the stimulus produces no congenital abnormalities in the usual sense, but a complete response of all the cells in the immature body – death.

A little later on, damage can be done to particular parts of the body as they develop. If they develop. If they are subjected to a harmful stimulus at a critical time of their division, fusion, or maximum growth, these processes may be slowed or completely stopped. Critical times for certain organs can be calculated:

	Weeks of Development						
	3	4	5	6	7	8	9
Spinal cord			—				
Heart			——				
Upper limb			—				
Lower limb				—			
Upper alimentary tract			—				
Lower alimentary tract			——				

These periods can be worked out in several ways. One is by discovering at what point in early pregnancy the embryo was exposed to factors which have constantly been associated with the subsequent abnormality of a given system. German measles is such a condition, and the discovery of its effect on the early embryo is an example of the value of retrospective surveys. Another research method is to expose pregnant animals to harmful agents at given times in their pregnancies and to assess the abnormalities after the offspring are born. While the experimenter must always bear in mind the warning given in the last chapter on animal work, this method may give a clue to the critical times of limb or organ growth.

If the mother should come into contact with harmful agents after these critical early days are over, no congenital abnormality is likely to occur, for the organ or tissue is already formed. Most organs are developed before the twelfth week of intra-uterine life, and the progress of the embryo after this is by growth only.

It is therefore obvious that the child is not at risk through the whole of the pregnancy but only during the first few weeks. If a pregnant patient were exposed to the fallout from an atomic bomb explosion during the first few days after conception, it is probable that the fertilized egg would be killed and passed from the body. Indeed the woman would bleed as the uterine lining was shed and probably would not know she had been pregnant. Should the explosion occur in the fourth week of pregnancy, the embryo might suffer a defect of its spine or spinal cord, such as spina bifida. Irradiation at the sixth week might arrest the development of a leg or of the rectum. If the bomb burst after the patient had reached the twelfth week, when the embryo would have been formed, probably no structural congenital abnormalities would be produced.

When we are considering the problem of abnormal babies we tend to assume that outside influences must all be harmful. In fact any physical factor occurring at a critical stage of development could theoretically do one of three things: improve the situation, leave it unaffected, or worsen it by killing or maiming the embryo. Many factors are arbitrarily assigned to the third group, whereas the vast majority of them in fact must fall into the first two; of these, the number that leave the embryo's situation unaffected must be the larger. Pregnant women are constantly in potentially harmful situations, yet the great majority of infants born are perfectly normal.

Irradiation

Penetrating rays can come from many sources. We are all subjected to cosmic rays from outer space. Some parts of the world have a high background irradiation from rocks and ores in the area. Cornwall has uranium ores mixed with the tin in the old mines; here the background level of ionizing rays is higher than in London. For a period of five years Russia and America tested their atomic bombs at intervals in the air and on the ground. This caused belts of fallout to pass around the world in the atmosphere, giving a temporary increase in irradiation. Bomb testing has now greatly decreased and is performed mainly underground; although the effects of the tests of six years ago are still measurable, they are greatly reduced. One of the commonest sources of irradiation in Britain is the diagnostic X-ray. Here a beam of X-rays is shone through the body from a generating source in a vacuum tube, to be picked up on a sensitized photographic film. It was estimated that until 1950 about a fifth of all ante-natal patients had an abdominal X-ray at some time in their pregnancy. This is no longer the case in Britain.

Experimentally it can be shown that a beam of high dosage penetrating irradiation causes cellular damage. There is no evidence of any beneficial or stimulating effect on body cells; all ionizing rays are purely destructive. Irradiation of a foetus in the uterus might affect the cell membrane, or the nucleus of the cell, having a long-term effect on the chromosomes, especially those in the gonads of the unborn child. The effect on the cell membranes is serious only where there are very big doses of irradiation, or if the cells happen to be vital links in a dynamic cellular growth system, as was discussed earlier. Here enzyme systems and molecular arrangements in the cells are upset, and this could lead to a congenital abnormality. The second or chromosomal effect would be unlikely to affect the foetus himself very much but could be laying down genetic defects for his children when he starts to reproduce in later years.

The possibility of producing alterations in the chromosomal pattern of future generations makes it essential that the whole population should receive the smallest possible amount of radiation. Added to this, the growth of the intra-uterine foetus in the first ten weeks of pregnancy may be stunted if the development of vital systems is interfered with by irradiation. Because of these risks, the general tendency in obstetrics in the late 1950s was to deplore diagnostic X-rays. As a result we remained uninformed about many factors in the mother's abdomen which could have been of immense value in caring for her in labour. The pendulum of opinion is swinging back, and now obstetricians are using X-rays where they are indicated and will help to resolve a difficulty. About one in twenty patients is so investigated. No one uses anything like as much irradiation as the experimental biologist does. Fewer exposures are requested and the improved techniques of radiology ensure much lower dosage than was previously required. Incorrect presentations of the baby and the narrowing of the mother's pelvis can sometimes be detected or made clear only with an X-ray, but the risks to the baby in such cases are much greater from a difficult labour than from the remoter dangers of irradiation.

Although not directly concerned with congenital abnormalities, another aspect of irradiation of the pregnant mother's abdomen should be mentioned, for it bears on the safety of the unborn child. In 1956 Dr Alice Stewart of Oxford suggested, on statistical grounds, that there may be a relationship between exposure to X-rays before birth and the later developments of bone-marrow disease in a child. Undoubtedly the cells of the unborn child divide rapidly and are unduly sensitive to the effects of irradiation. However, the risks of this type of damage seem small. It would appear that X-rays may be responsible for stimulating the bone marrow to become leukaemic in about one of 5,000 infants whose mother's abdomens were X-rayed during pregnancy. This is a small figure to balance against the number of deaths that would have occurred if the obstetrician had been kept in ignorance about the narrowing of the mother's pelvis. If only one of these latter were prevented, the proper use of irradiation would be justified. In fact, numberless infants are saved as a direct result of information obtained from X-rays. It seems on balance that X-rays, if requested only after due consideration by an obstetrician, are more likely to help in the delivery of a healthy infant than to give rise to the much publicized side effects that have worried mothers for the last ten years.

Diet

Before the Second World War, a large part of the population of Britain was too poor to afford a properly nourishing diet. When their womenfolk became pregnant, the grossly undernourished tended to produce a higher than average number of abnormal babies. It has been shown by experiment that in animals the deficiency of certain vitamins in the diet is associated with malformations. These facts are far from proving that the defects in the human population were definitely due to the dietary deficiencies. The pre-war women with malnutrition were of the lower social classes and many had an unfortunate genetic background. Their environment contained other factors that were known to produce malformations. As was pointed out before, the results of animal work do not of necessity apply to the human species.

No one is certain about the relationship of diet to the production of abnormal babies. In Britain, at present, nearly all the patients in the age-group liable to become pregnant are taking a well-balanced, perfectly adequate diet. The problem of other countries' populations, however, needs further thought. In Asia and Africa many people are on the borderline of starvation.

Congenital Anomalies

Acute Maternal Illness

When an acute infective illness occurs, the causative bacteria or the toxic substances produced by them pass in the blood to all parts of the body. In the case of a pregnant woman, these agents of disease may cross the placenta into the baby. He may get a form of the disease, but usually his mother's antibodies also flow into him and combat the infection.

If certain infections attack the mother in the crucial first few weeks of the baby's intra-uterine existence, congenital abnormality may result. Perhaps the best-known of these infections is German measles (rubella). This is a mild illness causing a temperature and malaise for a day or two. The patient usually has a headache and a stiff neck, accompanied by a faint rash on the face and trunk which lasts for two days. Commonly there is enlargement of the lymph nodes at the base of the skull. The majority of cases are uncomplicated; treatment is but a day in bed with aspirin and hot drinks. The spreading of the illness is not prevented by isolation of the patient, for it seems that the infectiousness is greatest before the rash appears, and therefore before the illness is diagnosed. Rubella is caused by a virus which enters the blood stream. It spreads across the placenta to the unborn child and may affect its development in the first twelve weeks of pregnancy. In 1941, an Australian ophthalmic surgeon first noted the correlation of cataract in infants' eyes with a history of maternal rubella during pregnancy. Heart disease and deafness are two other major complications.

It is hard to get figures of the incidence of congenital abnormalities following maternal rubella. Many workers have followed up large series both by the retrospective method (inquiring about the possibility of rubella infection in the pregnancy among others who have given birth to children with congenital abnormalities) and in the single-factor, prospective survey (following patients who contract rubella in the first twelve weeks of pregnancy and correlating this with the outcome). One of the most accurate of these series came from a London hospital, where the incidence of malformations was 7 times greater among children whose mothers had rubella in the first twelve weeks of pregnancy. In this group, congenital heart disease was 14 times increased, cataract 78 times and deafness nearly 40 times, compared with a group of control children whose mothers had not had the disease. Other surveys point to similar degrees of affection.

More difficult to assess is the prospective risk to an individual woman and her unborn baby. The variation of factors is enormous. Different people react to the virus in a variety of ways. The foetus is not of necessity more affected by a worse attack of rubella to the mother. The virus itself has a diversity of potencies, and different epidemics produce varying responses in patients. It has been calculated that the incidence of all malformations is 30–70 per cent for an attack in the first four weeks, 25–55 per cent in the second four weeks, and 20–40 per cent in the third four-week period. It is probable that after this time the effect of rubella on the developing foetus is negligible, but a few cases of deafness have been reported following infection in the fourth month of pregnancy.

Perhaps the best treatment in this instance is preventative. Once a person has had rubella, antibodies persist in the blood for a long time and usually give immunity for many years. Unfortunately, it can be such a mild disease that many women cannot recall having it. The very mildness of the condition makes diagnosis not very exact, and it may be passed off as a bout of flu. In some parts of the world, people take active steps to ensure that young girls get rubella in their teens, thus providing antibody cover for their pregnancies later. Australia, where the association between abnormalities and the disease was first noted, has set up 'rubella camps'. These are holiday camps where young girls can live for two weeks away from the rest of the community but in contact with the disease. Rubella is so contagious that it spreads rapidly through all the campers; it is so mild that it rarely spoils the holidays for more than a couple of days.

No such organizations exist in Britain, but any mother can see to it that her daughter comes into contact with rubella in childhood. Do not keep your girl away from a playmate who has German measles. Encourage them to play together. If your own child has the infection, let other mothers know so that they too can get their daughters' attacks over. Far better a couple of days of slight illness in childhood than the possibility of a harmful effect on unborn children. Unfortunately, social contacts like this do not always guarantee transfer of the disease. A surer method will be when an active immunization can be produced by injection of an inactivated strain of rubella.

Pregnant women should try to avoid contact with the condition if possible, especially if they have not had rubella in earlier life. The difficulty is that the stage at which the viruses may be spread is often reached before the sufferer knows she is ill. By the time the rash and headache appear, the condition is often no longer contagious. If a susceptible woman is accidentally exposed in pregnancy, a passive resistance can be given by the injection of antibodies from

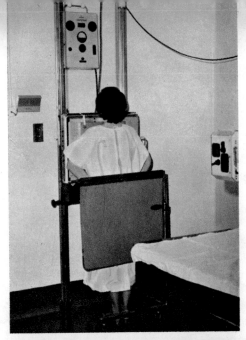

1. A pregnant woman having her chest X-rayed. Note the lead shields used to protect the growing baby from irradiation

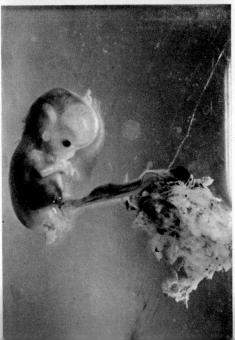

2. A foetus at eight weeks. Note the stage of limb and face development

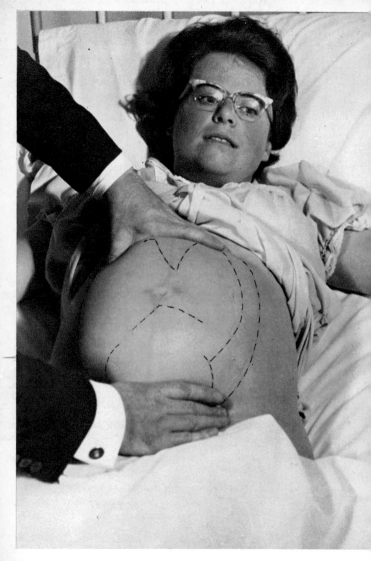

3. Palpation of the baby through the mother's abdominal wall

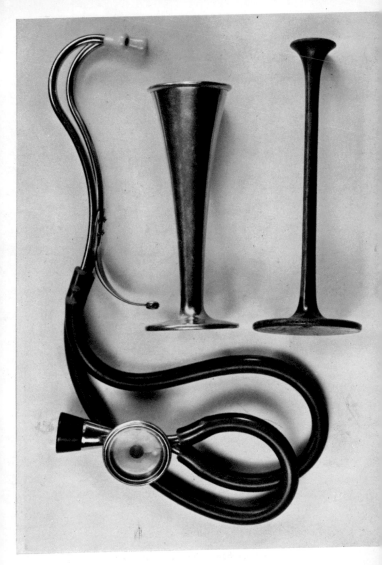

4. A modern stethoscope for listening to the patient's chest,
a monoauricular one for listening to the baby's heart, and an old-fashioned
monoauricular stethoscope that subserved both functions

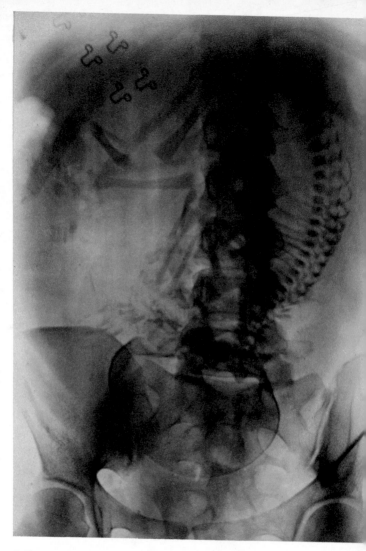

5. X-ray showing a normal baby in the uterus at about 36 weeks

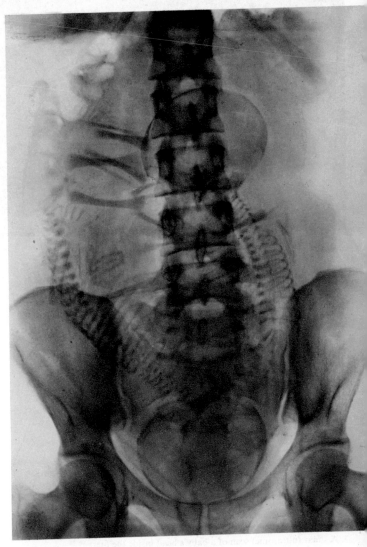

6. Twins in the uterus at 34 weeks. The first is lying with his head above the mother's pelvic cavity. The second is higher and presenting by the breech

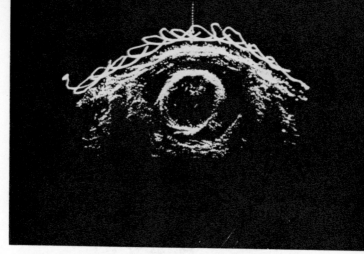

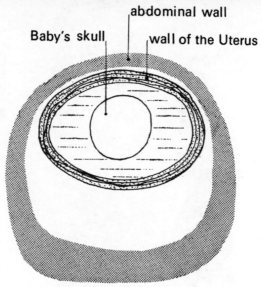

Baby's skull   abdominal wall   wall of the Uterus

7. A sonar (ultrasonic) scan of a baby's head inside the uterus

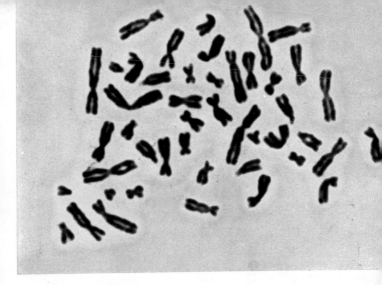

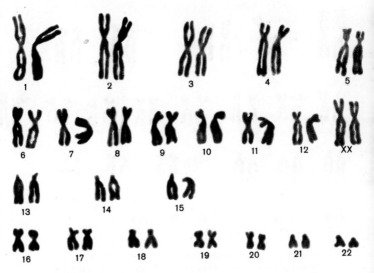

8. These are the chromosomes of a normal female. The genes that make up each chromosome are too small to be seen. In the lower picture the paired chromosomes have been arranged to show 23 pairs (22 numbered and 2x)

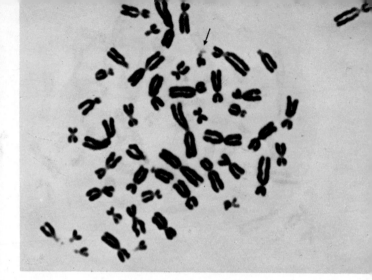

9. The Chromosome pattern of a child with Down's Syndrome. The arrow points to the extra chromosome which accounts for the physical and mental changes occurring in this condition

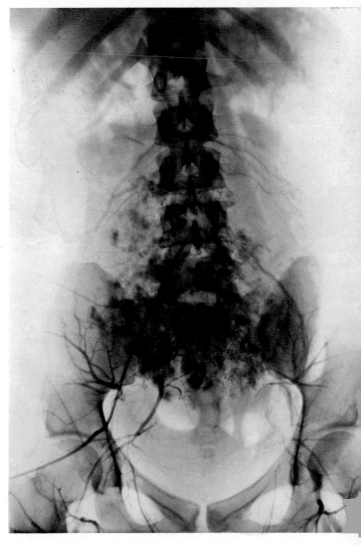

10. X-ray study showing the arteries supplying the uterus, the placenta and thus the foetus

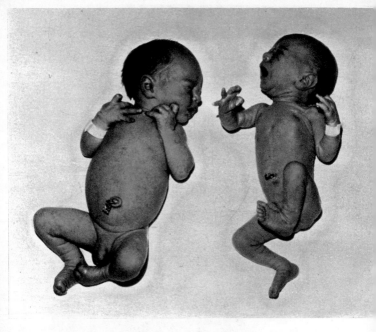

11. A premature baby on the right lies alongside a normal infant on the left

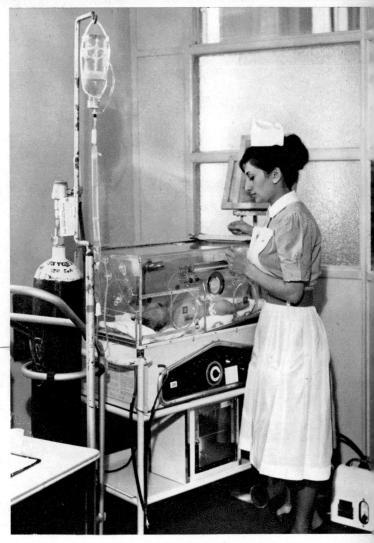

12. A premature baby weighing 4lb. 3oz. is being nursed in a special unit. He is being kept warm in an incubator with extra oxygen supply

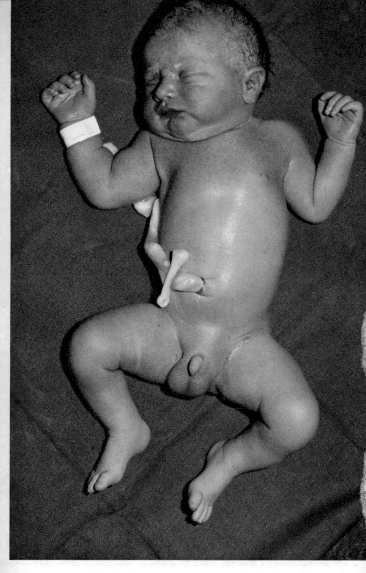

13. The baby of a diabetic mother. Note the podginess and thick skin folds

another person's serum: an extract is made from the blood of patients recovering from rubella, who have a rich supply of antibodies. This immunization may protect both mother and unborn child from the virus, provided it is given in time. Any pregnant mother who is in contact with a person suffering from German measles should see her doctor, so that he may assess the situation and order treatment if required.

Much discussion ranges now about the legal position of the termination of pregnancy. There are those who would lay down certain rigid indications for aborting a woman, and high on their lists are mothers who contract German measles. Under the 1967 Abortion Act, a doctor may advise interruption of a pregnancy on the grounds that the unborn child may have a substantial risk of suffering from an abnormality. The problem deserves dispassionate examination. Firstly, only in the first twelve weeks of pregnancy is the infant at maximum risk. Secondly, not all epidemics of German measles are equally virulent. The mother's response too is very variable and transmission of the virus across the placenta is not constant. Further, calculating from the most gloomy figures, over half the children may be perfectly normal and a substantial part of the remainder will have only minor afflictions. From this it can be seen that to destroy in the uterus a baby who stands a greater than even chance of being normal demands careful consideration. No all-inclusive law can be formed to cover all situations. Each patient should be considered individually. The wording of the new Abortion Act has not made it easier to reach a decision in these cases.

Other active infections have been cited as potentially hazardous to the infant in early pregnancy. Measles and malaria have been investigated. Both can produce bouts of high temperature, and these have been suspected of acting as non-specific factors at a crucial stage of embryonic growth. However, only marginal differences in the rates of congenital abnormalities are found when mothers with these diseases are compared with non-infected mothers.

The Asian flu outbreak in 1957 was investigated in Northern Ireland. A long-term prospective survey showed an increase in congenital malformations over the normal among the flu group. It is important to remember, however, the large numbers of healthy offspring born every day to the thousands of mothers who have had flu and other high-temperature-producing illnesses at any stage of their pregnancies.

Maternal Nutrition and Chronic Ill-health

An increased average income, a National Health Service and better standards of food in the last twenty years have reduced considerably the amount of chronic ill-health in the community, especially in the young people of the re-productive age-group. The pinch-faced, bowed, lame and halt of William Hogarth's drawings and Dickens' London are gone, and our ante-natal clinics are now attended by a group of women who have healthier bodies and better educated minds. Chronic illness is often rooted in malnutrition, and the two go together. As a direct result of improved nutrition, infant and maternal deaths in Britain have decreased.

The nutrition in a country is closely linked with its economic state, and both may be reflected in its infant mortality figures. Those countries with better standards of feeding have healthier mothers who produce healthier children.

Neonatal Mortality in Various Countries

(Deaths per 1000 live births occurring in the first 28 days of life. Taken from W.H.O. sources for 1961)

Yugoslavia	34
Portugal	27
Italy	23
South Africa (white population)	19
U.S.A.	18
Denmark	15
Great Britain	15
Australia	15
New Zealand	13
Norway	12

Confirming this view of the importance of nutrition, it is interesting here to note the figures given for two distinct populations inside a single country. In South Africa, while the infant mortality rate for the whites was 19 per thousand live births, comparative figures for the Asians and the Coloured in that State are 28 and 37. Other factors come in here such as attendance at ante-natal clinics and facilities available at labour. However, the nutritional background of mothers is a big factor in producing healthy babies. Since the Second World War this factor is much improved in Britain.

A woman with a long-standing illness often worries that she may not be able to conceive. Should she do so, she then fears that the child may be malformed. The problem of fertility is not within the province of this book, but it may be of comfort to know that the number of such reproductively crippling diseases is rapidly diminishing in the society in which we now live. However, the two factors cannot be entirely divorced, for the first is often the filter for the second; should, therefore, a patient with chronic illness become pregnant, she usually has a perfectly normal baby.

In this context it is important to differentiate between the chronic disease itself and the treatment of that disease as a potential hazard to the unborn child. An example will serve to explain this. There are no grounds for believing that the risk for a woman with thyrotoxicosis of bearing an abnormal child is increased over and above that of the general population. However, some of the drugs used for treating thyroid disorders might affect the infant. The importance of this differentiation is that, while the disease cannot be removed, the treatment of that disease could be altered and so any risk incurred could be lessened. It is this sort of analysis of cause and effect which might reduce the number of congenital abnormalities.

We shall now consider some of the long-term diseases that may affect women in the reproductive age-group.

Diabetes

Diabetes occurs in people of all ages, even occasionally in young children. Until the second decade of this century diabetic patients did not often become pregnant. Many died early, and the few who lived rarely married; of these many turned out to be sterile. The rare pregnancy resulted in abortion or a dead child delivered during a diabetic crisis. The discovery of insulin by Banting and Best in the 1920s altered this situation considerably. For the last forty years diabetics have been enabled to live nearly normal lives as long as they can keep up the body's supply of insulin by daily injections. Girls who develop diabetes in childhood now grow to be normal women and can safely marry and have children in the same way as their sisters. Recently, treatment of diabetes by tablets instead of by injection has been investigated; though as yet there seems to be little place for this type of therapy in the case of the pregnant woman, oral treatment does represent another breakthrough in the management of the diabetic.

The care of such patients in pregnancy is a very specialized aspect of obstetrics and should always be conducted in hospitals that have experience in treating pregnant women with diabetes. The many difficulties are dealt with in Chapter 13; only the aspect of congenital abnormalities is discussed here.

It seems probable that there is a slightly increased incidence over the average rate of abnormalities in children born to diabetic mothers. Possibly minor and unnoticed alterations of the maternal biochemistry in early pregnancy may account for this. Very mild attacks of low blood sugar (hypoglycaemia) might go unregarded by a diabetic woman who is vomiting, as many women do in early pregnancy. There is also some evidence that the bloody supply to the placental bed is altered in the diabetic state. The growing embryo's oxygen supply depends upon enough well-oxygenated blood from the mother arriving at the placenta all the time. If the arteries carrying this blood are narrowed, then at a critical time in development there may be relative oxygen shortage, with resultant deformities. Lastly, it is possible that a genetic element enters here, for diabetes has an inherited potential, and genes may be damaged by the metabolic upsets of the disease.

There is an increase in the number of malformations in the children of diabetic mothers, but many of them are minor. Ninety-four diabetic mothers in a hundred who produce living children will have perfectly normal babies. The small residuum have some abnormality, but many of these are not serious, such as accessory digits, and in no way affect the infant's life or health.

Chronic Urinary Disease

It is not uncommon in ante-natal clinics to meet women who have had long-term urinary infections. There is no evidence that this group of illnesses causes any increase in the congenital abnormality rate.

Tuberculosis

Tuberculosis is a disease now on the decrease in the age-groups seen in pregnancy. A slightly increased incidence has followed the immigration into this country of populations from poorer lands. The disease itself is not associated with an increase in rates of malformation.

Heart Disease

This is another illness diminishing in frequency in the age-groups of those having children. Here, too, the effects of pregnancy on the mother may be grave, but no congenital abnormalities seem to be due to her illness. The same can be said of *Epilepsy* and *Thyrotoxicosis*.

Cancer

The patients attending ante-natal clinics are usually too young to be affected by cancerous growths. Such a patient is rarely seen, but if she is treatment often must be started as an urgent measure to save her life. Many of the treatments for cancer can affect the unborn child (for example, powerful irradiation, or some of the strong drugs used to kill the actively growing cells). However, cancer itself does not cause any abnormalities in the infant. Hence if the treatment is delayed until after the twelfth to fourteenth week, it is probable that a normal child will result.

Mother's Age

So long as a woman is menstruating she will probably be producing eggs from the ovaries so that she still has a chance of becoming pregnant. Most children are born to mothers aged between 15 and 45. The author has delivered both a 13-year-old and a woman of 51, but these are exceptional. Two thirds of the children in Britain are born to women under the age of 30, and only 2.5 per cent (a fortieth) to mothers over 40.

It would seem that the woman who starts her family in her late teens or early twenties is most likely to produce healthy children. There is a slight increase in the number of abnormal babies born to the older age-groups. This increase in developmental abnormalities may follow the increasing number of eccentric chromosomal divisions that come with age. This, then, is really a genetic problem and represents another example of the difficulty in sorting out the causes of congenital abnormalities. The number of abnormal gene mutations occurring in the later years of reproductive life are above the previously quoted figure of 3 in 10,000; the chances of fertilization of an egg with an uneven genetic make-up are thus increased in the older mother. This increase is in fact marginal, and most mothers in their forties produce perfectly normal children.

Mongolism

One of the conditions that older mothers dread is mongolism. This is due to a chromosomal upset, and mongol infants are more commonly born to mothers over 40. The name is confusing, for the condition has nothing to do with any country in the Far East. The infants have a slight slit-ing of the eyes and the bridge of the nose is widened, which give an oriental look; hence the name. For the last decade, the synonym of 'Down's syndrome' is being used, for there is no racial suggestion here – the people of Mongolia have no monopoly of this abnormality. It would be analogous and equally incorrect to refer to all jaundiced babies as Chinese.

Down's syndrome is associated with the presence of an extra chromosome. Reference to Plate 8 shows that the normal human has twenty-two pairs of chromosomes, and one pair which determines sexual characteristics. The chromosomes are grouped according to their size and shape for classification purposes. Plate 9 is a similar plan of the chromosome from a child with Down's syndrome. The arrow shows that here, instead of a pair, three chromo-somes exist. This extra speck of tissue in the nucleus of each cell is responsible for all the changes that can occur. As well as the facial appearance mentioned above, the skin of the child is dry, and there are alterations in the creases of the hands and feet. Babies suffering from Down's syn-drome are very placid and their muscles have a low tone, so that the child feels limp when picked up.

This condition is usually detected soon after birth, and the child's development hereafter is slower than that of a normal child. These infants are very loving and affection-ate. They are behind their brothers and sisters in reaching mile stones such as learning toilet habits and dressing themselves, and they reach adulthood with a childish atti-tude to life. They are musical and often play instruments with zest, this being one of their pleasures. No one who has seen a child with Down's syndrome can doubt that he de-mands extra work and effort from the other members of the family; however, that same child is usually the most loving and loved member of that group.

The condition is not very common, occurring only once in every 800–1,000 births.

8 | Drug-affected Babies

Millions of women have produced millions of normal babies. Many such women have taken a whole pharmacopoeia of drugs in their pregnancies, and their babies have been quite unaffected. Very few patients thought or worried about this until the early 1960s, when the Thalidomide disaster was a reminder of the effects that drugs might have on the developing embryo. Here was a substance that was perfectly safe for the mother but, if taken at the critical time in pregnancy, had a tragic effect on the unborn child. Just after this episode, many other drugs were indicted as causing abnormalities; the majority of these treatments were quite safe, but immense worry was caused to mothers. At the time some pregnant women refused to take any tablets or medicines at all, thus exacerbating diseases that they had been suffering from for years. A wave of emotional hysteria followed, fed by uninformed comment from the popular press.

Once a drug had been blamed in this way, it was very hard to show it to be safe. In the last chapter it was shown how hard it is to prove cause and effect in these matters. An example demonstrates this point. Just after the Thalidomide troubles, a letter appeared in a medical journal reporting ten abnormal children born to mothers who had taken Ancoloxin, a drug which combats the nausea of pregnancy. A few days later, a Swedish Board of Health article seemed to show a similar fact. These two events were blown up, so that the drug seemed in the minds of thousands of people to be as bad as Thalidomide. Many patients were taking these tablets at the time, for it was one of the best treatments for reducing vomiting in pregnancy. Immediately, many of them stopped their treatment, and other patients refused to start. The second group had only to put up with their nausea and vomiting, but those who had actually been treated for several weeks before the scare started were in a worse predicament: they too stopped the tablets, but they were left with six months of worry until their children were actually born, for they were frightened that they might have harmed their babies. The episode produced a great deal of mental ill-health, some of which may still be apparent today.

In fact, both reports, if appraised scientifically, were unsound. The ten cases covered a large range of abnormalities. There was no pattern, no one malformation that was associated with the taking of the drug; nor was any exact time relationship established. The background population from which these ten cases were drawn was not examined. At the time, this anti-vomiting drug was possibly the commonest prescribed in pregnancy, and the ten cases of abnormality could well have appeared by chance. The Swedish series was similarly suspect on statistical grounds. A year later, after further, more balanced work, the report was contradicted, but the second announcement received very little press coverage, for it had not much news value. It took four years to conduct a properly prospective survey on this drug. The results of this trial, published a few years ago, cleared the drug from blame. Much unhappiness and worry had been unnecessarily engendered by uncritical comment on a subject that was not clearly understood.

In the last chapter we said that any external influence on the pregnant woman could improve the total situation, leave it unchanged, or worsen it. We also concluded that most ante-natal influences came into the second class. But when we are considering the influence of a drug, we run into difficulties. Spontaneous abortion in the early stages occurs often because of the abnormality of the developing embryo. This is Nature's way of eliminating an undesirable type and of keeping the species healthy. Some drugs can be used in early pregnancy for the purpose of inhibiting the contractions of the uterine muscle, thus reducing the likelihood of the evacuation of the uterus, the mechanism of abortion. It follows that the final effect of a group of such drugs might be to cause the retention of abnormal embryos, and the drugs would then appear to have been responsible for the malformation of the babies subsequently born.

Not many drugs do act in this way, but this is another example of wrong deductions being drawn from a group of facts.

How Drugs Act

The ways in which drugs cause abnormalities in the embryo are not definitely known in every case. They may cause some alteration in the mother's body which indirectly affects the child in the uterus. Certain drugs, for instance, affect the pituitary gland, and changes in the output of this gland might have an oblique effect on the developing child. This is not a very likely mechanism; but it is known, on the other hand, through experimental work on animals, that removal of the adrenal glands in the pregnant female sometimes causes reabsorption of the embryo.

Another possibility is that the drug affects the diffusion rate of oxygen and foodstuffs across the placenta. If this were to happen at a critical point in the development of the embryo, its growth could be affected. It is known that in animals certain hormones can have this effect.

Most drugs act on the embryo directly, by passing through the placenta and arriving in the embryonic blood. Since this passage by diffusion depends on the size of the molecule, it is obvious that drugs with smaller molecules will more easily penetrate the placental barrier than those with large. Diffusion continues until an equilibrium is established between the maternal and embryonic blood; usually this equilibrium exists while there is a slightly lower concentration of the drug on the embryonic side. Some drugs are, however, differentially concentrated, and in these cases they are present in larger amounts in the embryonic blood. In this category come some of the drugs used in the treatment of cancer, and it may be that it is the high concentration in the embryo's blood stream which accounts for the abnormalities seen in foetuses after exposure to these drugs.

So many interrelated factors come into the causation of developmental malformations that it is difficult to pin down any one drug as a cause of trouble. If it consistently produces grossly unusual defects, as was the case with Thalidomide (which caused the absence of arms or legs), it is not difficult to identify, but this is an exceptionally clear-cut example. Equally it is difficult to prove the converse, the innocence of a drug. No drug can be said to be absolutely blamefree, for we do not know the cause of many abnormalities. Over 400 drugs have been shown to affect the foetuses of animals in experimental work. Before automatically extrapolating these results to the human infant, species differences, proportional dosages, and relative stages of pregnancy should be considered. This was stressed earlier. In fact only a handful of drugs have been observed to be closely associated with the production of malformations in human beings. In the brief review that follows, these recognizably harmful agents are discussed. Others which have been under investigation in the past are also examined. Many have been shown to have no obvious effects; a few must remain still with their guilt 'not proven'.

Antibiotics

Antibiotics are one of the most commonly prescribed group of drugs in our society. Perhaps the patient has a chronic infection and is on long-term therapy, or there may be an acute inflammatory condition arising *de novo* in pregnancy. The second situation demands the drugs as a medical emergency; the first might be precipitated into an acute flare-up if administration of the previously prescribed antibiotics is stopped, and this could be more dangerous to the safety of the unborn child than the drug itself. In fact all antibiotics have been thoroughly tested and are used only when shown to be safe. They all cross the placenta and are useful for treating infections of the unborn child while it is in the uterus.

Tetracycline was the centre of a controversy a few years ago, when limb and mouth malformations were reported in chickens after the parent hens had been fed on it. Reference to the original experiments shows that the hens had received about fifty times more than a pregnant woman would ever be given as a therapeutic dose, and only at this high concentration was there retardation of bone growth. Experiments on other animal species do not show this to happen in all species. Pregnant rats were given over

1,000 times the relative dose that the pregnant human mother would get, and no abnormalities resulted. A species sensitivity is implied here. Millions of women have taken tetracycline in pregnancy; if it caused abnormalities this would almost certainly have been noticed by now.

Tetracycline does have one disadvantage, however. Given in later pregnancy it sometimes causes a yellowing of the child's bones. This is not serious except in the one place where bone shows in the body – the teeth. Probably only the milk teeth are affected, but there is some evidence that, as well as being discoloured, the tooth enamel is less resistant than normal, and so caries may start earlier in life than usual. It is possible that certain types of tetracycline affect the teeth less than others, and if it is necessary to prescribe this group of drugs, doctors usually choose those which are potent but with which there is less risk of giving rise to undesirable side effects.

Streptomycin is an antibiotic often used for the treatment of tuberculosis. Usually the treatment has to go on for months in order to cure the infection, and should pregnancy occur, it must continue, for the disease may flare up at this stage. Alarms were raised in the early 1960s when it was reported that streptomycin caused deafness in unborn children. When traced to its source, this report proved to concern four children in Europe who were born deaf to tuberculous mothers. The dosage of streptomycin given to these mothers was much greater than anything we use in treatment in Britain, and, further, there was a history of deafness in two of the mothers' families. Since then the subsequent histories of large numbers of mothers attending chest clinics and receiving streptomycin have been followed up, and there is no evidence of an increased incidence of deafness among their children.

Congenital Anomalies

Sulphonamides are safe chemotherapeutic agents and have not been connected with the subsequent appearance of any congenital defects. If their mothers have been given certain sulphonamide preparations in late pregnancy, some infants may develop transient jaundice, but this usually fades in a short time with no further bad effects.

Steroid Hormones

Cortisone is being used effectively for an increasing number of conditions. It is life-saving in adrenal diseases, asthma and some bowel ulcerations, and there has been an enormous increase in the amount prescribed over the last ten years. Steroids are given usually in two levels of dosage, depending on the state of the patient's own cortisone production. Some diseases (for example, tuberculosis or cancer) destroy the adrenal gland, where these steroids are made. Sometimes surgeons remove both glands to help disease in other parts of the body. Both situations leave the patient with no source of internal cortisone manufacture, and treatment with cortisone must then be given to make up for this. Replacement dosage aims at imitating the normal physiology of the body and so small doses are used. Patients receiving this treatment are usually beyond the pregnancy age-group and so do not come into this discussion. Those few younger women who are receiving this treatment usually produce normal children, and there is no evidence that dosages of a size calculated to replace the normal physiological output cause foetal abnormalities.

Additive or pharmacological doses may be much bigger; they are given in addition to the cortisone made by the mother's own adrenal glands (although there is evidence that after treatment has lasted some time the natural production of cortisone is damped down). Such treatment is often required in the reproductive age-group and has given rise to fears that it will cause congenital abnormalities. The risks have probably been exaggerated. It is true that a large volume of work has been done which shows that cleft palates can be produced in the offspring of animals if they are given large doses of cortisone in pregnancy, but this could be an example of the species differences mentioned earlier in this book. If pregnant mice of certain species are fed cortisone at a dosage equivalent, weight for weight, to that which would be given to a human, cleft palates appear very commonly in their litters. The same dosage does not affect a pregnant rabbit's offspring; increases in cortisone up to fifteen times as much have to be given before any effect is noted. From comparative figures it appears that the mouse, the rabbit and man are three species with increasing resistance to the effects of cortisone in pregnancy.

In 1958 much alarm was caused by reports from Central Europe of cleft palates following cortisone treatment. When details of a large number of patients on cortisone were reviewed, the situation came into perspective. Out of 322 pregnancies where a reasonably high dosage of cortisone had been used, three children were born with a cleft palate or hare lip. All three came from the same area, where a group of ten women had been treated with a very high dosage of cortisone. In this whole series, a ratio of three to 322 is more than random variation, while three out of ten would be obviously significant. But this is not taking into account the family and genetic background of the ten women. There may have been inherited tendency to non-

111

union of the two sides of the palate in embryonic life, for cleft palate is often a familial trait.

Since these early reports, thousands of women have been safely delivered of normal infants after cortisone treatment. The incidence of cleft palate after the use of cortisone in pregnancy appears to be low. Owing to the character of the underlying diseases, the treatment is usually of a long-term nature. It starts long before the pregnancy is initiated and is in progress when fertilization occurs. In accordance with the 'all or none' law quoted earlier in this chapter, if the dosage is too high the whole embryo will be killed at a very early stage before the organs have started to form. Thus an abortion follows rather than local malformations. Usually the dosage used is much less, weight for weight, than that in animal work and the human foetus does not seem very sensitive to the lower levels of concentration. Lastly, if cortisone is being given, it is usually for a fairly serious condition, and treatment must continue irrespective of the pregnancy. Cortisone must not be stopped suddenly; it must be withdrawn gradually, or the body will react in a very violent fashion. The time required for gradual reduction of cortisone dosage, if this were medically permissible, might in any case overlap the vital first few weeks of pregnancy during which the diagnosis is often uncertain.

There are many practical disadvantages to the discontinuing of cortisone treatment in pregnancy, and every patient must be judged individually. No exact figure can be given of the risks, for there are too many individual variables (why the cortisone was used, when it was used, how much was used and all the other considerations that concern the pregnancy). It can be stated, however, that those who continue on the usual dosage given in Britain stand 'much less risk of its affecting their unborn children than was previously feared.

Progesterone is one of the hormones made by the ovary and, in pregnancy, by the placenta. It helps to keep the uterus in a relaxed state for the retention of the growing embryo. Occasionally women are taking progesterone tablets for other reasons when they become pregnant. A few patients are progesterone-deficient and are sometimes given this hormone in early pregnancy to try and make up for the lack of natural product. Both these groups of women may have an extra amount of progesterone, and they do run a slight risk of producing minor alterations in their infants. If certain types of progesterone are used, a female infant in the uterus may get external signs of masculinization. A male infant is unaffected, so half the unborn children are not at risk. The alterations in the female are only at the external level. Internally a normal uterus and ovaries still develop, but the external genitalia appear masculine – the clitoris slightly enlarged and the lips of the vagina incompletely separated. In consequence there may be some doubt as to the sex of the child at birth. Occasionally, if the parents are not aware of this problem, such children may be brought up as boys. Should doubt exist, simple chromosome tests can be done on the blood and on cells from the lining of the mouth. These will give an answer as to the true sex and will help to differentiate these cases from sex aberrations from other causes. Correcting the minor but confusing external signs is a simple matter of plastic surgery and can easily be done in the first six months of life. The girls grow up quite normally after this.

This may seem to be a serious trouble for the infant, and it may be wondered why we use such drugs at all. Firstly, a woman may inadvertently become pregnant while taking progesterone; she would know nothing about the pregnancy for a few weeks and so the very immature embryo would be exposed to its effects. Secondly, a large body of evidence is accumulating to show that some women who might otherwise abort can be stopped from doing so. The baby resulting from this successful pregnancy may be male and therefore unaffected, but if it is female, surely it is better to have a live baby with a minor, correctable blemish than no baby? Perhaps more important now is that research in the last seven years has produced a type of progesterone which has the desired effects in stopping the miscarriage without masculinizing effects on female embryos. This is the form of this hormone that doctors now usually prescribe in early pregnancy.

Here is another drug that produced a scare in the uninformed. 'It changes their sex in the womb' was an expression used by one patient. The preceding paragraphs show that this remark is not true; the risk is small and the correction easy. Probably, with more doctors using the newer progesterone products, the risk has now been removed.

Anti-cancer Drugs

Cancer-curing drugs are rarely required in the child-bearing age-group, but where they are in use a serious illness is being treated and so the treatment must continue. The author has delivered normal babies from women who have been treated with several of the more commonly used anti-cancer drugs, but the risk of abnormalities is higher in these cases than in the rest of the population.

One drug in this class deserves particular attention. *Aminopterin,* usually given in the treatment of leukaemia, was used by doctors therapeutically and by the lay public criminally to induce abortions, for it is powerfully toxic to the unborn child. In about half the cases it has the effect of killing the baby and precipitating an abortion. At other times, given in the same relative dosage, it does not quite do this: instead of killing, it maims, and the damaged baby goes on developing in the uterus, to be born months later with congenital deformities. This drug is very toxic to the mother too, and patients who take enough to cause abortion or mutilation of the foetus are often seriously ill with the side effects: they become anaemic, and the number of white cells in the body is lowered. It is therefore not a reliable abortifacient, and if it fails leaves a living but malformed baby. It is never used in obstetrics now.

Anti-thyroid Drugs

Patients in the reproductive age-group are often under treatment with these drugs. Over-activity of the thyroid gland (thyrotoxicosis) sometimes requires medical treatment to damp down hormone production. The drugs used for this purpose can cross the placenta and, rarely, interfere with the mechanisms of the foetus's glands. In an effort to overcome this, the baby's thyroid may increase in size, thus leading to mechanical troubles at delivery. Usually the gland recovers quickly after birth and all is well in later years. This problem is dealt with in Chapter 13.

More recently, thyrotoxicosis has been very successfully treated with radioactive iodine isotopes. The thyroid gland actively takes up iodine from the blood; if some of that iodine is made radioactive the gland will still absorb it avidly and store it. Thus the gland will be irradiated by sources inside itself and its over-active state will be damped down. All irradiation is destructive; hence very careful calculations must be made of the exact dosage of I_{131} required to destroy just the correct amount of the gland. If this isotope were to be given to a pregnant woman, the baby's thyroid would take up the radioactive iodine just as the mother's would, for the placenta presents no barrier. This would then have severe effects on the baby's thyroid, destroying vital glandular tissue, sometimes even to the extent of leading to cretinism. Radioactive iodine is therefore rarely used for women below the age of forty-five, and never if there is any suspicion of pregnancy.

Thalidomide

Thalidomide was first made in 1954. It was available from 1956, being widely used as a safe sedative drug, prescribed by doctors for those who could not sleep. One of the difficulties about allowing patients to have large numbers of barbiturate sedatives is that they may take an overdose, accidentally or by design, and this might lead to death. Thalidomide had the advantage in that ten to fifteen times the usually effective dose could be taken and the patient would still wake up the next morning.

Before Thalidomide was first marketed, the pharmaceutical company in Germany which patented it tested it on animals and performed controlled human trials. The drug passed these examinations, being shown by the tests then in use to be safe, and millions of doses were prescribed in Western Europe. It was used for men, women and children, for it seemed so safe. Some obstetricians recommended it as a sedative in pregnancy, since it seemed to produce fewer hangover effects the next day than the barbiturates. At children's hospitals too it was popular, for the smaller dose tablet fitted snugly into a well-known 'mint with a hole'. This was taken by the children with no fuss. For the men, the children, and the women who were not pregnant, this safe drug had no hidden dangers.

However, some women in early pregnancy were taking Thalidomide, and to their unborn children this was unexpectedly dangerous. In 1958 a child who had no arms or legs was born in West Germany. She was noted as a congenital abnormality. Her deformities aroused no suspicions: the absence of limbs (amelia) is not an unknown malformation, though it is rare. Sporadic instances of the condition occurred, and in November 1961 a paediatric medical meeting was held in Münster at the Children's Hospital, at which thirty-four infants with abnormalities of the arms and legs were presented. Dr Lenz of Hamburg suggested there might be a relationship between this large number with unusual abnormalities and the fact that their mothers had taken Thalidomide.

At this time Professor R. W. Smithells had noticed, on examining his survey of congenital abnormalities in the Liverpool region, five such cases of limb abnormalities in a year. Again it was the unusual nature of the malformation that drew attention to these infants. The German report came in at about this time, and quick checking back in Liverpool showed that all the five mothers had taken Thalidomide in early pregnancy.

Reaction to these researches was rapid. Within nine days the drug was withdrawn from the German market, and by fourteen days all sales had stopped in Great Britain. The firm manufacturing Thalidomide made every effort to see that every doctor who might use their product was warned of the possible dangers. No more Thalidomide was prescribed, and patients were urged to return any surplus tablets from medicine chests and bathroom cabinets.

Action came commendably quickly, but because of the necessity for speed the public had to be told of the suspicions. Anxiety spread, and at ante-natal clincs many worried women wondered if their unborn children would be affected. Although they had stopped taking Thalidomide, damage to the infant might already have been done. One of the worst aspects of the affair was that all those mothers who had been at risk had to wait, and wonder, for six months or so before they produced their babies. Ultimately some 800 affected children were born alive in England and 2,800 in West Germany

Thalidomide was never widely sold in America. At the time it was under review by the Food and Drug Administration Department. This was fortuitous, for the investigations had nothing to do with congenital abnormalities. There had been reports of bizarre nervous side effects in those who took large quantities of Thalidomide. These patients had tingling in the fingers and cramps in the legs, while their finger-nails became brittle. In consequence, the drug had not been released for general use, which was most fortunate, for in the Americas sedatives are used even more than in Western Europe.

The effects of Thalidomide on the unborn child are now well known. The absence of the long bones of the limbs brings the deformed hands and feet close to the trunk, giving the flipper- or seal-like look to the child. The external ears may be malformed, and birth marks are common on the upper lip. Internally, there may be abnormalities of the heart and kidneys, and the gall bladder and appendix are often affected too.

Without doubt Thalidomide causes malformation of the unborn child if it is taken at any time between the thirty-seventh and the fiftieth day (5–7 weeks) after the last menstrual period. These thirteen days are quite specific. Cases of abnormal babies have been reported after the taking of only one dose. No cases of damage to the brain were reported, although such developmental defects are relatively common among most malformed children. The drug is thought to have no effect on the chromosomes or on the genetic future of any patient. This means that the only pregnancy to be affected would be that during which Thalidomide was actually taken.

The story of Thalidomide has been told in detail. No pregnant woman will take this drug again, and so this particular group of drug-affected babies will not be produced again. The episode was, however, important, for it brought home the possibilities of drugs harming unborn infants while the mother was quite well. Had the abnormalities been of a more commonly produced nature (for example hydrocephalus), the detection of the cause would have been even harder and would have taken much longer. Fortunately the outbreak was confined, but it acted as a stimulus to research and surveys which have already increased our knowledge of congenital malformations and their prevention.

Anti-vomiting Drugs

Vomiting accompanies the early months of pregnancy in two thirds of women, but fewer than one per cent are severely incapacitated. Despite this, women are offered drugs to relieve this condition at the very time when the possibility of external events affecting the embryo is at its greatest. It is most difficult to assess the effects of anti-vomiting drugs at this stage; until recently no one could tell if there was any risk at all.

Occasionally anti-vomiting medicines are blamed for abnormalities. The obverse, however, should be considered. Could not the effects of vomiting on the woman's biochemical state be the prime disturbing factor? Even more basically, could it be that women who vomit have some inborn variation of their metabolism that might be associated with the production of abnormalities? These two theories have been under discussion for years. It is unlikely that the last is true, for many women vomit and few produce affected infants. In relation to the first theory, it would be expected that the degree and number of the abnormalities would bear some relation to the type of vomiting and the subsequent biochemical alterations in the mother's blood, and again this does not seem to be so.

Earlier in this chapter we mentioned the problems that arose when a widely used anti-vomiting drug, Ancoloxin, was suspected of being a cause of abnormalities; it was impeached by two reports within a short time, and soon was widely believed to cause abnormalities in babies. It was shown that neither report was substantiated, but it was difficult, even so, to prove the drug's safety. In a London teaching hospital, a group of 75 women given Ancoloxin in early pregnancy produced 5 affected babies, while 60 similar women not so treated had 3 babies affected and 3 abortions. Another group of 369 women was examined, all of whom had had the drug: only 2 produced children with congenital abnormalities. These were both retrospective surveys. To mount a prospective survey with this drug as the prime factor obviously requires time. The results of such a survey were reported in 1964 by Professor Smithells at Liverpool. Here 220 women were followed through pregnancy, Ancoloxin having been given in the first twelve weeks. Two children only were born with congenital defects, which is less than the random variation.

The drug was first prescribed in 1955; if it had indeed had a deleterious effect on the foetus, an increase in the incidence of malformations would by now have been discovered. In fact for three years about ten per cent of pregnant women in Britain took the drug during the early stages of pregnancy, and there was no increase in the number of abnormal babies born during that time.

Vomiting in early pregnancy is a miserable business. Nowadays it rarely makes anyone seriously ill, but it can cause a great deal of unhappiness and disruption of normal domestic arrangements. It is right that relief for this symptom should be offered, but only if that relief can be shown to be safe for the unborn child, who is particularly at risk during this time. A few drugs have been shown not to be associated with the production of abnormalities and these should be used for treatment. Any new drugs produced should of course be tested thoroughly before being used.

Other Drugs

Insulin is used for treating diabetes. Although it was suspected in the scare years of the early 1960s, there is no evidence that this drug is linked with the production of abnormalities.

The same clear assurance cannot be given about the oral anti-diabetic drugs *Tolbutamide* and *Chlorpropamide*.

Congenital Anomalies

Both have at times been suspected in connexion with foetal abnormalities, but more recent, larger surveys have not confirmed any such association. It must be remembered that the underlying disease being treated (diabetes) is itself a factor in congenital malformation. These two drugs will probably be proved safe in the next few years, but at the moment of writing they are in the not-proven group, and it would be wise not to start a patient in the first weeks of pregnancy on such treatment.

Aspirin has sometimes been blamed in connexion with the production of abnormalities. The evidence is based on animal work. If doses of 300–900 mg./Kilo (that is $\frac{1}{200}$-$\frac{1}{100}$ of an ounce for every pound of body weight) are fed to pregnant rats it harms them. Some of the rats die, others produce abnormal litters. The dose used is somewhere in the region of 150–200 times that which a pregnant woman would take in pregnancy. Indeed, she, like some of the rats, would probably die of aspirin poisoning before being able to give birth to any infants, normal or abnormal. Aspirin is probably the commonest patent medicine taken in Western Europe. There is no real evidence that it causes foetal abnormalities.

Nicotine is only one of the chemicals that come in tobacco smoke, but it is one with strong effects on human tissues. The pharmacology of tobacco smoke is complex, as recent research into the cause of lung cancer has shown. Nicotine in its pure state can cause animal abnormalities if given to the pregnant animals in large enough dosage. These amounts are far greater than any smoker would obtain by absorption from the lungs.

There is another aspect to cigarette smoking. Mothers who smoke heavily in pregnancy (more than twenty cigarettes each day) produce smaller children. Differences between smoking and non-smoking mothers are of course more than just a cigarette between the lips. The social background tends to be different; temperament, nervous tension, eating and drinking vary with the cigarette habit, and any of these could influence the size of the infant. Surveys have been conducted in which everything but the smoking habit is matched in several groups of mothers, and they have shown that at full term the babies of heavy smokers are several ounces lighter than those of non-smokers.

Even if we accept the idea that smoking affects the unborn child, the problem is not as simple as that of giving a drug in pregnancy. Drugs can often be stopped or others substituted, but to stop an addicted smoker is a different matter. Even if she were made to give it up (and this is in itself a large therapeutic problem), the nicotine poisoning might be replaced by mental tensions, alterations in eating habits and variations in digestion. These in their turn might have more effect upon the unborn child than the low dosage of nicotine alkaloids to which the mother's body is probably used.

That heavy smoking has an effect on the infant's size is undeniable. If, therefore, the mother can voluntarily and without anxiety cut down her cigarettes for the duration of pregnancy, she will be helping to build a bigger infant.

This chapter has discussed the effects of drugs on the development of the embryo. Methods of investigation have been shown, and the effects of certain medicaments have been detailed. Over 400 drugs have been alleged to affect the litters of pregnant animals if given in large enough doses, but of these only half a dozen have any known effect on the human species; the rest have been shown to be reasonably safe.

This can be said with hindsight. What of any new drug? Neither animal work nor clinical trials seemed to show up the toxicity of Thalidomide, and it was on the market for a few years before its dangers were realized. Now, all countries test new drugs on pregnant animals as part of their preliminary safety trials, and so one more safeguard is provided. However, trials with Thalidomide showed that most species of pregnant animals were unaffected, only the New Zealand white rabbit responding as the human species so unfortunately did; so even these recent experiments with animals cannot be regarded as conclusive.

In Great Britain a Committee was appointed by the Government in 1964 to check all new drugs. After pharmaceutical firms have made a new product, it is submitted to the Dunlop Committee for consideration. The Committee has three functions. It advises whether a new drug should be submitted for clinical trials, whether it should be released to the public, and thirdly it studies any adverse effects reported, in relation to established drugs already in common use. Physiologists, pharmacologists, physicians and pure scientists investigate it fully, and only when they are satisfied of its safety is it released for use. This screening is thorough and a safeguard to all users of drugs in Britain.

Those who have read this chapter carefully will have noted that no drug can be completely cleared of a low incidence of association with abnormalities in the unborn. We do not know the cause of most malformations, and, until we do, every alteration in the mother's body must be suspect. Many drugs seem to be safe because of the millions of times they have been used without harmful effects; most doctors feel, however, that no drug should be used lightly in early pregnancy. If there are medical indications for treatment, then a well-established pharmaceutical preparation is given. Doctors are aware of the risks involved with each drug; it is from the medical profession only that medicaments should be obtained. One of the difficulties in investigating the Thalidomide episode was that many of the mothers in Germany had bought the tablets without a prescription, or else had taken tablets prescribed for another member of the family. No one should ever take a medicament prescribed for someone else. When doctors give a drug to a patient they are thinking of all the factors that affect that individual. These factors may be very different for another person.

The developing embryo is tough. Considering that all mothers are exposed to a large number of chemicals, food additives and medicines, remarkably few infants are affected. With careful ante-natal management, such drug-produced abnormalities are becoming rare, and much unhappiness could be avoided if mothers realized that the baby in the uterus is not so unprotected as they think. He is resilient, and after the first three months of pregnancy is most unlikely to be influenced by any outside source of trouble.

The Prevention of
Congenital Malformations

Much is written nowadays about the control of the number of children born into this world; less thought goes towards influencing the quality of these babies. Those who
have read the previous chapters in this section will realize
how little we know about the causes of deformities in the
unborn child. All the factors already recognized among
these causes occur in only a small proportion of all the
pregnancies that result in abnormal children. Since we are
so ignorant about causation, it is difficult to consider the
treatment, or, what would be better still, the prevention, of
these factors. This chapter deals with those causes that are
understood, for each year medical research reveals a little
more of the picture.

In the last two decades, the figures for newborn infants'
deaths have not dropped greatly in Western Europe, and a
constant proportion of these deaths results from errors of
development. Much has been achieved in the rehabilitation
of such deformed children as survive, but preventing the
deformity occurring in the first place is much more difficult. The problems of prevention are now considered in
the same order as the causations were.

Genetic Factors

People generally marry because they have fallen in love.
Usually this is a chance phenomenon, although the chances

of meeting and falling in love with any one person are obviously increased if the two people involved are of similar society, class, interests or working habits. Once two people have fallen in love they will rarely accept advice to separate on medical grounds. Hence as a means of preventing congenital disease, medical refusal to sanction a marriage is more a theoretical than a practical idea.

Perhaps more acceptable would be advice to use contraception sensibly. The ethics of contraception are a matter of individual religious or moral belief, but its logic is a community matter: those who are liable to produce abnormal babies can avoid doing so by preventing the joining of defective ova and sperm. One of the most firmly entrenched ecclesiastical opponents to contraception has recently been rethinking its policy in Rome; pronouncements made in the summer of 1968 saddened many who were hoping for a change of the Roman Catholic Church's philosophy. But among people who accept it, contraception is obviously one of the most effective ways of preventing the birth of abnormal babies.

An extension of the reasoning behind this idea is sterilization. Here the advantages of higher success rates are coupled with the disadvantage of the irreversible nature of this form of contraception. If the tendency to produce abnormal babies is a genetic one, it is permanent, and the grounds for the contraceptive method being permanent also are strong. The defect may occur in either partner. It must be remembered, however, that not all marriages are permanent. Death and, more commonly in the marriageable age-group, divorce cannot be dismissed as impossible. Hence, although it is the woman who is usually presented for sterilization, it should logically be the partner who is responsible for passing on the damaged genes who should have the operation. The suggestion of male sterilization has always caused shocked looks and shudders from men. They fear loss of potency and virility, ignoring the scientific fact that neither occurs. The large bulk of semen is made in the prostate gland, only the spermatozoa being added from the testicles. To operate on the male is easy, takes only fifteen minutes, and can be done on an out-patient with local anaesthesia. The tube on each side that leads the semen from the testis to the penis is divided just under the skin in the groin. Female sterilization involves opening the abdomen and tying the Fallopian tubes. This is a bigger operation, requiring a general anaesthetic and ten days' stay in hospital.

Some abnormal offspring come from genetically defective parents who are mentally retarded. These are the families in which sterilization could offer help, for mentally subnormal parents are often unable to understand contraceptive techniques. However, in the present state of the law, surgical procedures such as sterilization demand the patient's consent, and mentally defective parents are not in a position fully to comprehend and give such permission.

Recent changes in the abortion law in England authorize yet another weapon in the battle to prevent congenital malformations. If, in good faith, two doctors think that 'there is a substantial risk that if the child be born it will suffer from such physical or mental abnormalities as to be seriously handicapped', they may consider terminating the pregnancy. The mothers who may be considered under this heading are those with a strong genetic likelihood of producing abnormal babies and those who have been exposed in early pregnancy to recognizedly dangerous agents. The first group would require expert genetic counselling to assess the risks of producing further abnormal infants. This science is in its infancy, and often the lack of previous follow-up information makes deductions invalid. The second group of mothers are slightly easier to assess, for something is known of the effects on the foetus of a number of agents. There are, however, many difficulties here; the problems of advising the mother who has had German measles have already been mentioned (page 93), and while we do know about the certain effects of a number of drugs, there are difficulties in assessing new drugs, as was mentioned in Chapter 8. The new law will undoubtedly bring relief in its train, but it does not solve the problem of deciding what is a 'substantial risk'.

Environmental Factors

Alexander Hamilton, a Scottish obstetrician, in 1780 advised pregnant women 'to lead a regular and temperate life, their company should be agreeable and cheerful, their exercise moderate, especially in the early months when the connexion between the ovum and the womb may be feeble'. This is the sort of good advice that is still offered nowadays at the ante-natal clinic. Most women, however, do not attend the clinic until ten to twelve weeks of pregnancy, by which time, readers of this section will remember, the risk of most congenital abnormalities will be roughly over. It is therefore important that every woman should be aware of the problems of very early pregnancy and take intelligent action accordingly.

In Britain, ante-natal care is part of the National Health Service and is free. Probably many women come for advice and attention earlier than they would otherwise do because of this. Undoubtedly, in a society that pays for its medical care, the higher the income of the patient's husband, the earlier in pregnancy her ante-natal care starts. Some doctors think this practice should be taken further even under the Health Service and suggest that for the good of tomorrow's society women should be paid to attend pre-natal clinics earlier in pregnancy than they do. At the time of writing (1968) the maternity grant is £22, payable at twenty-eight weeks of pregnancy. It has been suggested that either an additional sum should be paid to those who produce certification that they attended a clinic before the sixteenth week of pregnancy or the grant should be split. In France, two ninths of the grant are available before the twelfth week, four ninths before the twenty-fourth week and three ninths by the thirty-sixth week. A similar system could be introduced in Britain. Educating patients is the most important and probably the best way to effect earlier ante-natal care in the long term, but it is slow and will influence only a certain number of women. Monetary reward would help to bring in just those women who tend to disregard medical advice.

In the early ante-natal period, factors known to be harmful should be guarded against. Abdominal X-rays are avoided, and chest X-rays taken only with proper precautions, as was mentioned earlier. It is probable that the amount of irradiation used in diagnostic radiology is in any case too little to affect the unborn child, but this is not absolutely certain and so the abdomen is protected. All the drugs that are suspected of causing trouble should be eschewed. It has been stressed that no drug can be said to be completely blameless; in addition to this, women sometimes do not realize they are taking drugs. Anyone swallowing two tablets after every meal would recognize this as drug-taking, but this seems not to apply to the woman who puts nose drops in each nostril or to the heavy smoker. A rational approach must be used here. Drugs given for serious conditions must be continued, but starting fresh treatments or using new drugs should be avoided at this time. Obviously a woman in early pregnancy should avoid contact with those who are known to have German measles or acute infective illnesses. However, only when we can stop all people from contacting rubella can we stop pregnant women from so doing. Prevention by previous infection and the resulting immunity is the important step; even better will be an active immunization against German measles. Vaccination against smallpox should be avoided unless there is a real risk of the disease. All other infections should be treated vigorously, for the foetus might respond badly to rises of the mother's temperature.

Results

Most of the advice given above seems pretty negative; mainly laying stress on the avoidance of various risks. On the whole there is little positive action one can take to prevent abnormalities occurring. In the last year or so, however, diagnostic horizons have been pushed back, and, with more accurate knowledge of what is happening inside the uterus, slightly more active steps can be taken. Already the sex of the unborn child can be accurately predicted by an examination of the cells in a sample of amniotic fluid drawn off from the uterus. Thus forearmed, doctors can confidently discount the presence of certain sex-determined familial diseases where the baby is of the sex not affected by them, and so they can reassure many mothers before the child is born. An example of this would be the case of a woman with several haemophiliac children, whose amniotic cells predicted a female child, for haemophilia affects only males.

With certain conditions this process can go further. In Chapter 5 we saw how certain genetically determined diseases were reflected by the chromosomes in the nucleus of the cells. These chromosomal changes can sometimes be detected in cells floating in the amniotic fluid. Thus, a sample drawn off in very early pregnancy could be examined for these mutations; if any were found, the mother could at least be given more accurate information about the potential future of her unborn child and advised accordingly.

It may be that we shall never completely eliminate congenital abnormalities. The measures mentioned in this chapter, and others that future research may uncover, will reduce the numbers, but under the natural laws of species variability a certain number of abnormal babies will be born. Genetic counselling can help to cut down the number of babies born to high-risk parents, and ante-natal care will ensure that factors known to be harmful are avoided and so 'the blots of Nature's hand ... such as are despiséd in nativity' will be lessened. To do this much is the everyday business of ante-natal care. To strive to improve upon it is one of the great challenges to obstetric research.

3 | Intra-uterine Hazards

One of the basic requirements for the continuation of life is oxygen. This gas must be supplied to all living plants and animals whether they are in space-craft thousands of miles from the earth or in the depths of the sea. The absence of life as we know it on the other planets of our solar system is attributed to the lack of oxygen in their atmosphere. On this earth, animals are divided into those who obtain oxygen through their lungs (air breathing) and those who get it dissolved in water through a gill system (water breathing). A few reptiles have a third method of absorbing oxygen into their blood, via their moist skins. The air breathed in by adult mammals, of which humans constitute one species, contains twenty per cent oxygen. This is taken down into the fine sacs that form the surface of the lung and there the oxygen dissolves in the moisture lining these membranes. The dissolved gas then passes into the blood contained in small vessels that line the lung sacs and is pumped by the heart to all parts of the body. Every cell requires oxygen to live, but some that work more actively than others require a higher proportion. Even the living cells in the middle of hard bone require some oxygen but obviously not as much as a cell in the leg muscles of someone who is walking. This differential requirement is often adjusted by the volume of the blood flow to the different types of tissue and cell. The bones have a small blood supply, the leg muscles a large one. If a person trains as an athlete, and so uses the muscles more than usual, blood vessels enlarge and provide an increase in blood flow which brings the cells the extra oxygen they require.

The child before birth has no direct access to the air. He is entirely dependent on such oxygen as he can extract from his mother's blood. Figure 17 shows how the blood is

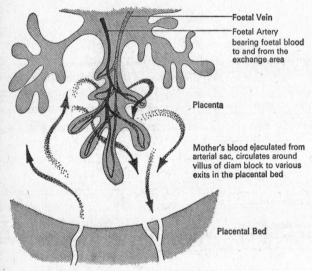

Foetal Vein

Foetal Artery bearing foetal blood to and from the exchange area

Placenta

Mother's blood ejaculated from arterial sac, circulates around villus of diam block to various exits in the placental bed

Placental Bed

Figure 17. A villus, bathed by the mother's blood. Here exchange of oxygen and food stuffs occurs from mother to baby.

pumped along the aorta, the main artery of the body running down the back wall of the mother's abdomen (see Plate 10). The aorta branches several times, and one of the last arteries given off is that to the uterus. This vessel runs up the side of the uterus, and one of its major branches goes to the area of placenta. Behind the disc of placental tissue, the mother's blood forms a lake which bathes the surface of the placenta. This surface area is greatly enlarged by numerous finger-like processes which contain the embryo's blood vessels and are covered by a very thin membrane (Figure 18). Oxygen dissolved in the mother's

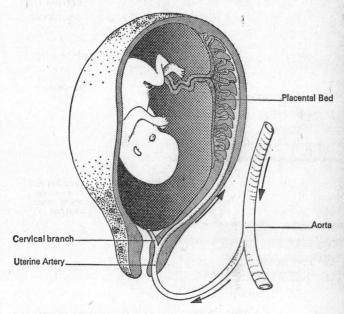

Figure 18. The blood supply of the placenta.

blood is thus able to diffuse into the baby's blood quite easily, without the two blood streams coming into direct contact. Once the embryonic blood is oxygenated, it is driven by the action of the foetal heart along the umbilical cord from the placenta to the baby's body.

The unborn child lives in an environment of lower oxygen concentration than either that of the mother or that which he breathes after birth. In order that he may survive and grow actively in this relatively low oxygen state, various adaptive mechanisms come into play. Living surrounded by liquor in the uterus, the unborn child is kept at a constant temperature and so little energy is required to keep up body temperature. His total energy requirements are low, and therefore the oxygen need is less. Certain organ systems are not used, and so their blood supply is small compared with that of the newborn infant. Blood is shunted away from the unexpanded lungs and by-passes the unused alimentary tract, while the actively growing brain has a large blood supply and is kept well oxygenated. The oxygen itself is mostly carried in the blood in a loose chemical combination with the major blood pigment, haemoglobin. This pigment has a complex molecular structure, but the haemoglobin that is present in foetal blood is different from that in the adult: it can take up more oxygen and so be a slightly more efficient transport mechanism. Another adaptation to oxygen lack is a biochemical adjustment which can take place in the cells of the developing infant. The tissues can temporarily build up an oxygen debt, performing their functions in a modified way that can for the time being do without oxygen. Like all debts, this must be repaid and, like financial ones, often with interest.

Despite all these adaptive mechanisms, the infant in the uterus is at risk when oxygen levels fall. A careful examination of stillborn infants showed that a third of the deaths were caused by lack of oxygen. While some of these changes may not have been the primary cause of death following as they did in the wake of other factors, the deprivation of oxygen would have aggravated any pre-existing situation. Such oxygen shortage can occur at three levels, maternal, placental or foetal.

Maternal Causes

The embryo's oxygen supplies depend upon an adequate supply of well-oxygenated blood from the mother. Some women have respiratory diseases so that the efficiency of the lung surface for absorbing oxygen is impaired. Others suffer from diseases of the heart which cause the adequacy of the pumping mechanism to be impaired so that the oxygenated blood is not efficiently sent to the tissues. Both these groups of diseases often result in the patient showing cyanosis – a blue tinge to the lips and extremities. The blood arriving at the uterus in these patients is deficient in oxygen.

Some women are anaemic in pregnancy. Good ante-natal care checks this point and provides preventive and curative measures to cope with it. In some underdeveloped countries, however, it is not unusual for pregnant women to have a blood concentration of the iron compounds that carry oxygen which is only one third that of normal. Under such conditions the oxygen-carrying power of the blood is greatly reduced and so the infant is at peril.

The major vessels that bear blood may be constricted so that the flow rates are reduced. This is common in later life but rare in the reproductive age-group. The placenta lies with one surface bathed in a pool of maternal blood, which is brought from the uterine arteries to the placental bed by smaller vessels. Some conditions cause narrowing of the small vessels so that the placenta is presented with a poor blood supply. This happens when the mother suffers from raised blood pressure, either antedating the pregnancy (hypertension) or occurring only in pregnancy (pre-eclampsia). There is evidence that some other maternal diseases, such as diabetes, may also affect the placental bed vessels. These changes are of a chronic nature, and so the embryo is living at a constantly lowered oxygen level. In the steady state, the adaptive mechanisms mentioned previously can cope, but the foetus is not fitted to stand any extra stresses added to the long-term one. For this reason patients with raised blood pressure are advised to rest and are often brought into hospital. The elevation of blood pressure is often too little to cause serious worry about the mother's condition, but it does give warning of an increased risk to the unborn child. Strict bed-rest may help the situation by allowing a relatively increased blood supply to the uterus. This enables the infant to grow a little larger so that he is better equipped to stand labour and delivery.

Other measures have been tried to improve the situation. Some obstetricians believe that lowering the blood pressure may prevent the alterations in the placental bed vessels. Here cause and effect may be difficult to elucidate. In some parts of the world, abdominal decompression is carried out with the same hope. The mother is enclosed up to the armpits in an airtight chamber or bag from which air is evacuated intermittently. This subjects the lower part of the body, including the growing uterus, to a lowered pressure, usually nine tenths of atmospheric pressure. Claims have been made that this 'flushes out' the small placental bed vessels and so prevents the situation described above from happening. That this method produces larger and more intelligent babies is also claimed. The technique is an experimental one and its effects are being tested in various centres in Britain. So far no very strong evidence has come to light that the blood flow to the placenta increases, but, as with every new idea, this method needs full and critical evaluation before final opinions are expressed.

During labour the uterus contracts regularly. These muscular efforts are weak, short and irregular at first, but as labour becomes established the contractions become stronger and last up to a minute each. During this muscular squeezing, the blood supply to the placental bed is cut down. The blood vessels travel in between the muscle bundles that make up the thick wall of the uterus and are squeezed during each contraction. This obliteration of fresh blood to the placenta lasts thirty to sixty seconds and usually can be accepted by the normal well-adapted infant. If, however, he is in oxygen debt for some other reason, contractions sometimes depress him even further. This is reflected in alterations in his heart rate. As a check on such possible changes, frequent observations of the foetal heart are made in labour. The obstetrician can then take any such signs into consideration and act in good time to effect a safe delivery of the infant.

Placental Causes

The placenta is the growing embryo's lung. If it is inefficient, then oxygenation of his blood is reduced and the sequelae may be serious. Sometimes the cause of trouble is obvious. In certain conditions, often associated with pre-eclampsia, the placenta becomes separated from its bed in the uterus by active bleeding between the two. This can be serious for the mother and the child and should be met by hospital treatment, utilizing blood transfusions and sometimes an operation. Occasionally the placenta is embedded by chance in the lower part of the uterus. This area stretches greatly in later pregnancy and should the placenta be attached there it may get stripped off. In this case also there

141

is bleeding behind the placenta, depriving the infant of some of his oxygen supply. Both these conditions may be associated with a loss of blood from the vagina and should a patient have such a symptom in late pregnancy, medical advice should be sought immediately. Prompt treatment may save lives in the early stages; if the symptoms are neglected, the results can be serious.

A large group of longer standing causes of placental inefficiency exist and are not properly understood. Pre-eclampsia has been mentioned already as affecting the blood vessels of the placental bed. The same condition may also cause changes to the membrane separating the foetal blood vessels in the placenta from the pool of maternal blood. At the beginning of this chapter it was stated that oxygen could diffuse across this membrane, which in later pregnancy is only one cell layer wide. Pre-eclampsia is associated with a thickening of the membrane so that the membrane width is increased by several cells. This can act as a barrier and slow down oxygen diffusion.

All tissues in the body age. Most are continuously being renewed and last us a lifetime, but the placenta is needed for nine months only and its ageing process can be proportionately short as is its life. There is evidence that when the pregnancy is unduly prolonged senile changes occur in the placental vessels and membranes, again adversely affecting the transfer of oxygen.

From the placenta, the re-oxygenated blood runs in a vein back to the infant. The vein is bound up in the umbilical cord with the arteries, and along this lifeline the circulation of blood between the placenta and the embryo occurs. Blockage of these vessels can harm the child, for it cuts off oxygen. Very rarely, a knot could occur spontaneously in the cord. This is most likely to happen very shortly before delivery, and the child is usually born before any serious harm has been done. Sometimes loops of the cord can get twisted around the infant's limbs or head. Provided they are loose no harm follows, but if they tighten they may affect the blood flow. Again such events rarely occur until birth is imminent.

When the membranes surrounding the baby rupture in early labour, a gush of the fluid that has been cushioning the infant escapes into the vagina. If the baby is not right down in the mother's pelvis, its head blocking the mouth of the uterus like a ball blocking a plug hole, a loop of umbilical cord may be carried down with the liquid so that it is dipping down into the vagina. Provided this cord is kept warm and moist no immediate harmful effects follow. Should cooling occur, or labour contractions nip the cord between the pelvis and the baby's head, the vessels may be sent into spasm. This condition, prolapse of the cord, is constantly guarded against in obstetric practice, for if it is diagnosed in good time the baby can be delivered safe and well.

Foetal Causes

The proper oxygenation of the unborn child depends upon an intact circulatory system which can transfer the oxygenated blood from the placenta to the various parts of the body. Rarely there are congenital abnormalities of the baby's heart or blood vessels that interfere with blood flow. If they are very severe, the infant may not be able to stand the added stress of labour and may perish during delivery. Even less frequently, he suffers from severe anaemia, which is discussed in Chapter 11. Such conditions produce a relative oxygen lack in the foetal tissues, but other than these, there are few causes of anoxia in the unborn infant.

Although not strictly within the compass of this book, it should be mentioned briefly that some factors in pregnancy and labour can give rise to asphyxial troubles in the infant after delivery. Among these are some of the pain-relieving drugs, which, if given in labour, can affect the control of respiratory powers in the newborn. For this reason, obstetricians carefully gauge such drugs if they are given to the mother in the last hours before birth. Should a patient progress more rapidly than was expected, measures can be taken to reverse the depressive effects; skilful watch is required to ensure that this is done.

Many of the causes of asphyxia are preventable. As this chapter has tried to show, good medical care is constantly watching for these causes and dealing with them in good time to prevent trouble. Child-bearing is essentially a normal process. The aim of ante-natal supervision is to keep it so.

11 | The Rhesus Problem

During millions of years of evolution, the human species has produced people who are distinguished from each other by having blood of different groups. To mix these groups is dangerous, for the blood clots on contact. In consequence, the blood of anyone who has to have a blood transfusion must be checked against the donor blood to establish that both are of the same group. Pathologists can identify the group by testing a small sample of the patient's blood against the serum of a known group. If clotting occurs, the blood must belong to a different group and should be re-checked until the correct serum is found. The most common types of blood are those classified as A, B, AB, and O, and it is to this last group that most people's blood belongs. Over and above this system of grouping, and unrelated to it, is the distinction of blood into two other categories, Rhesus positive and Rhesus negative – the term Rhesus is used because the difference between these two kinds of blood was first discovered in the Rhesus monkey. Eighty-five per cent of the population of Britain are Rhesus positive, while the remainder are considered negative, for they have no Rhesus antigens.

The Cause of the Problem

As was mentioned in Chapter 6, all familial traits are carried in the genes of the chromosomes. Two genes, one from each parent, determine each characteristic of the child. These genes may each contain the same instructions to the future cells – for example, both may be for blue in the case of eye colour, and here there would be no question as to the colour of the child's eyes. If, however, one gene has the instruction 'blue' and the other 'brown', the result may be a compromise, as, say, hazel; or one gene may have the supremacy of command and overrule the instructions contained in the other gene. In the example given above, brown is usually 'dominant' over blue, and the child will have brown eyes. The genes involved with the Rhesus factor of the developing child act in the same way, and here there can be no compromise. Since the Rhesus positive genes are always dominant, the blood of the child can be Rhesus negative only when both the genes from mother and father are Rhesus negative. But the child's blood will be Rhesus positive if only one parent supplied a Rhesus positive gene. It is not therefore surprising that the majority of the population are Rhesus positive.

Apart from during pregnancy, no problem exists: should a blood transfusion be required the groups of the patient and the donor are matched for the Rhesus factor and no trouble ensues. But the situation is different where the two bloods are those of a mother and her unborn child. Whilst a Rhesus positive mother is likely to produce a Rhesus positive child, thus avoiding any difficulties, the child of a Rhesus negative mother may have the same Rhesus group as a father who is Rhesus positive. (There is a fifteen per cent chance of his being Rhesus negative too, in which case all is well.)

It happens sometimes that a few of the baby's blood cells escape across the placental membrane and enter the mother's blood stream. Should these cells be Rhesus positive, they act as foreign agents and provoke the formation of antibodies in the maternal blood. This protective reaction does not harm the mother: she is Rhesus negative and the antibody is lethal to Rhesus positive blood cells only. The antibodies can, however, diffuse back through the placental membrane into the baby's circulation. There they attack the foetal blood cells, which are Rhesus positive, destroying them and releasing their contents.

If this reaction continues for long the foetus becomes anaemic, and breakdown products of the haemoglobin from the foetal red blood cells collect in the tissues. Sometimes vital brain centres are stained, giving rise to neurological symptoms, and the infant has a pale yellowish skin colour.

The Rhesus factor becomes a problem in about one out of every two hundred deliveries. All women have their Rhesus group checked at the first ante-natal visit. Should it be negative, a watch is kept for the production of antibodies. It is rare for any of the baby's blood to leak into the mother's circulation before mid-pregnancy. It then takes a little time for antibodies to be formed, and so no tests are needed until the 30th to the 32nd week of pregnancy. If any antibodies are present, a second test at 34 or 36 weeks indicates whether or not their production is increasing.

The length of time required for the production of antibodies makes it rare for a mother to make any significant amount of them in her first pregnancy. Although the infant's cells can leak across at any time from mid-pregnancy onwards, they commonly do so in quantity only during delivery and especially during the separation of the placenta after the baby's birth. This is too late to affect the baby then being born, but it may act as a stimulus for antibody formation during the next pregnancy.

In Great Britain sensitization during a previous pregnancy and delivery is the commonest cause of antibody formation. It is possible, of course, that before the discovery of the Rhesus factor in the 1940s Rhesus positive blood might have been given by transfusion to Rhesus negative women, who would then have had an even more potent stimulus towards antibody production. Nowadays very strict precautions are taken to prevent this happening.

When the Rhesus negative woman becomes pregnant for the second time, she may again bear a Rhesus positive infant, and may already have antibodies present in her blood. Renewed production of these antibodies is now quicker, for the antibody-forming tissues have been sensitized previously. In consequence, more antibodies may be made earlier in pregnancy, and they may pass across the placenta and affect the baby.

Commonly the first affected child is not very seriously anaemic or jaundiced. With good care, no more than observation, with blood checking, is required, and no active treatment is necessary. Subsequent pregnancies may stimulate greater and earlier antibody formation so that a more dangerous situation can arise for the unborn child. Anaemia and jaundice may be much more severe and imperil life. Since the child is exposed to antibodies all the time he is in the uterus, the logical treatment is to remove him from this noxious atmosphere as soon as possible. It is in the last four words that the problem lies. If he is delivered too soon, the problems of prematurity and immaturity are great; should he be left too long, he may perish as a result of the antibodies' action in his blood. The exact timing of delivery is a difficult task, and in order to judge it correctly the obstetrician requires as much information to help him as he can get.

The situation for the mixed Rhesus marriage is, however, by no means desperate. Not in every placenta do red cells leak from the Rhesus positive baby to the Rhesus negative mother; perhaps one or two such pregnancies may pass without sensitization. This would mean that the antibodies produced for the first time in the third pregnancy of a Rhesus negative mother are probably not going to have any effect on the babies until the fourth pregnancy at the earliest, by which time many parents will feel that their family is complete. A further factor is that forty per cent of Rhesus positive men can produce a Rhesus negative baby; these men are known in genetic terms as 'heterozygous': their chromosomes can carry one – the dominant – gene for the Rhesus positive factor, and one for the Rhesus negative. About half their sperms, therefore, carry one gene and half the other. It follows that in forty per cent of 'mixed' marriages – those in which the mother has Rhesus negative and the father Rhesus positive blood – roughly half the children born will receive the Rhesus-negative-carrying gene from each parent. These children will be Rhesus negative themselves and incur no danger in the uterus: antibodies in the mother's circulation from a previous stimulus do not threaten the baby who has no Rhesus positive blood cells.

Not every succeeding child is going to be more seriously affected than his elder brother or sister. The impression that the Rhesus problem worsens with each pregnancy is incorrect. The risks certainly can become greater in the second than in the first affected birth, but they seem to even out somewhat after this, so that each pregnancy tends to have the same chance of a successful outcome, rather than a diminishing one.

The Treatment

Our major treatment of mothers affected by the Rhesus problem has up to the present been to remove their infants from the environment of the antibodies at the correct time. All Rhesus negative mothers who are at risk should be cared for and delivered at a hospital which is used to dealing with Rhesus blood groups and babies that may require treatment. This may mean a fair amount of travel for the pregnant mother to attend ante-natal clinics at a strange hospital in the next town, when she would rather visit her own family doctor around the corner. For the safety of her unborn child, the journeys are essential. Only by accurate checking can some guide to the infant's progress be obtained.

Several factors influence the obstetrician's decision about when to deliver the baby. The state of the previous children at birth and the increase in the level of antibodies in the mother's blood are two important ones. Some specialist centres gain assistance in this problem by taking a small sample of the liquor around the baby. This gives an indication of the level of the breakdown products from the blood cells which the infant is excreting. In experienced hands this can be a most useful factor in assessing the extent to which the baby is affected.

At some point in later pregnancy, it is decided that the infant is big enough for delivery. Further growth in the uterus would be at the expense of increased risk from Rhesus antibodies. Labour is then induced; most mothers of this group have had babies before and so the delivery usually follows soon after induction and is moderately speedy. Immediately after birth, the baby is carefully examined and his blood tested. His Rhesus group is checked, his degree of anaemia and the level of blood breakdown substances estimated. The results of these tests may indicate that the infant is only mildly affected and so he needs only to be kept under observation; the tests are re-checked in a few hours, for the antibody from the mother is still circulating in the infant's blood. Although no new antibody is crossing now into his blood stream, that which is present can still act, although less potently.

Some infants are more severely affected at birth. They may be obviously pale, and jaundice may follow very soon after delivery. The tissues may retain fluid so that the baby looks puffy. Such an infant requires urgent treatment. His blood must be washed out and replaced with fresh Rhesus negative blood with no antibodies in it; this further removes many of the blood's breakdown products. Obviously, one cannot drain the child of blood and then fill him up again, as though emptying a garden pool in the spring to scrub it out. Instead an exchange transfusion is performed: a little blood is removed at a time and is immediately replaced by unaffected blood. In this way, the infant's blood volume is kept constant. To continue the analogy, it is like replacing the water in a garden pond that has gold-fish and plants in it: a little clean water is trickled in at one end while the dirty water is tapped off at the other. The pond cannot be emptied because of the fish and plants, and so replacement is not quite as efficient as by the complete clearance method. So, in exchange transfusion, much but not all of the affected blood is removed. Occasionally, an infant still has so much affected blood in him that a second exchange is required; this can be done a day or two after birth.

Mention was made earlier of the effects of the bile pigments on the brain. In Chapter 2, the evolution of the brain was discussed, and here it was seen how the cerebral cortex (the higher, or thinking, brain) evolved above the midbrain (lower, or subconscious, brain). In the latter are collections of nerve cells that regulate vital functions of the body such as respiration and blood pressure, body heat and muscle tone in the limbs and body. It is in this region that a large amount of bile pigments might act deleteriously. If these groups of nerve cells are damaged biochemically, the infant's body is affected. Should the brain cells be involved, the child would be irritable and might have fits, while the limbs and back would become tense and rigid. This spastic state need not be permanent, but nerve damage could occur at this stage; careful watch is therefore kept on the infant's blood so that an exchange transfusion can be performed long before the levels of bile products reach these dangerous heights. This type of spasticity is very rarely seen now, for good paediatric care prevents the condition occurring.

The Future

Our means of dealing with the Rhesus-affected baby at present are centred around protecting him from the antibodies and replacing his blood when he is born. To accomplish the first of these, measures are in hand to help the infant to live safely in the uterus for a further few weeks in order to achieve the delivery of a more mature child. One method, developed in New Zealand, is to provide the affected infant with Rhesus negative blood while he is in the uterus. With X-rays as a guide, a long transfusion needle is led into the unborn child through the mother's abdominal wall (a local anaesthetic is given first), her uterus and then the baby's skin, and Rhesus negative blood is given to the infant. This staves off anaemia for a week or two longer to give a larger and so more mature baby at delivery. Intra-uterine transfusions like this require much skill, but are being given in several centres in Britain with good results.

The ultimate aim in treating Rhesus-affected babies is either to prevent foetal red cells crossing the placental membrane into the mother's blood, or to prevent the formation of antibodies. The first is difficult, but certain obstetric procedures are known to be associated with a higher foeto-maternal blood leak, and should be avoided if possible. The second line of blocking or preventing antibody formation is being actively pursued in laboratories all over the world. In the lead here is Liverpool, where Professor A. C. Clark has developed a blocking serum which will very soon be available to all Rhesus-affected women. There is an old principle in immunology that the stimulating factor (antigen) does not cause the body to respond with the production of its own antibodies if there are antibodies already present. Now that the antibodies to the Rhesus positive factor have been isolated, they can be given to the Rhesus negative woman at the time when she is most likely to be exposed to the red cells from the Rhesus positive baby in the uterus. These outside antibodies will prevent the formation of the mother's antibodies, but will not survive long enough to affect the child in any subsequent pregnancy. At present this procedure is still being developed, but within the next year or so it will be perfected; Rhesus negative women will be able to receive this protective treatment at each pregnancy and the problem of severe jaundice and anaemia in the Rhesus positive baby will have been solved.

In this chapter, only the Rhesus problem has been discussed. Several rarer blood groups can act in a similar fashion to the Rhesus factor, but have their own specific antibodies. The problems posed by them can be guarded against too, and the children they affect can be treated. Very few women are affected in this way each year in Britain.

All in all, only one in two hundred pregnancies is affected by the Rhesus problem. Of these, over ninety per cent of the children born are treated and respond well, to become perfectly normal children. Once the first days after birth are surmounted, and the antibodies absorbed away, no further trouble will occur. The Rhesus problem is being overcome at present by vigilant ante-natal care, demanding the mother's cooperation, and by skilful paediatric treatment of the newborn. The future lies in the research of the immunologists, and within a few years protection will be available to prevent this problem occurring.

12 | Prematurity

The British Perinatal Mortality Survey was mentioned in relation to maldeveloped babies in Chapter 5. As well as studying fully every delivery occurring in Great Britain for a week in March 1958, the investigation continued for a further three months, sifting the facts about every baby who was born dead or died in the first week of life (the perinatal deaths). Much valuable information came from this inquiry, for it was the first time a thorough scrutiny of these points had been made on a nation-wide scale. Among the facts which emerged was the prevalence of prematurity. A half of all the deaths were associated with prematurity, and, while it might not have been the only or even the major factor, it is commonly an exacerbating factor in many other causes of death in this age-group.

The Premature Infant

A premature infant is one weighing less than $5\frac{1}{2}$ pounds at birth. This definition was laid down by the World Health Organization and accepted by all member countries of the United Nations in 1948. It has the merit of being easily understood and applied. Anyone who can read a weighing scale can make the 'diagnosis', and so statistics can be gathered simply. Its drawback is its all-embracing nature. Into the net are drawn many perfectly mature children who happen to be a little lighter than usual but who may come of small stock; escaping are a larger group of bulky, but immature, infants whose bodily behaviour in the first days of life demands expert attention but who may not get it, for they are not technically premature.

To criticize the standard definition is not to be able automatically to suggest a better one. More important than the infant's size is the maturity of the way his body functions, which would be a better criterion for assessment. Probably the system which must above all others be working properly is the brain. Life depends upon this organ's ability to maintain heart and respiratory rhythms, to keep a steady blood pressure in the body, and to balance heat production against heat loss, so stabilizing the internal temperature. The assessment of all this is the skilled business of paediatricians who have specialized in the physiological study of the newborn. Sometimes laboratory tests help, but in the end the diagnosis must be based upon a doctor's opinion. How much simpler to read a pair of scales. Opinions vary here, as in any other scientific field. In any case, there are not enough experts to go round, and so this method of estimating true immaturity cannot be used.

Another straightforward way of assessing maturity depending on a simple measurement, might be based on the length of time that the infant developed in the uterus: if he is born early he is obviously 'premature'. But when the length of pregnancy was discussed in Chapter 3 it was noted that a number of women (fifteen per cent) have variable menstrual cycles, so that dating a pregnancy is likely to be inaccurate in these patients. If the length of the pregnancy can be calculated accurately, an infant is considered to be immature by gestational age when born before the thirty-eighth week. However, because of the uncertainties of the length of any one pregnancy, this would not be a satisfactory universal working delineation; the weight definition is still the most useful, provided its drawbacks are remembered.

Plate 11 shows a premature baby beside a mature one. As well as the obvious smallness, the wrinkled skin will be noted, for the premature infant has very little fat, which leads to rapid heat loss. Perhaps as striking as these appearances is the difference in behaviour. While the mature child wakes for feeds at intervals, bawling loudly if not satisfied very soon, the premature infant is perpetually half asleep and has a weak cry, like a small cat mewing. When given a feed he sucks badly or not at all.

Causes of Prematurity

One in ten children in England is born before the thirty-eighth week. Of all babies, seven per cent weigh less than $5\frac{1}{2}$ pounds at birth. Many patients go into spontaneous labour some weeks before pregnancy might be expected to end. We do not know what starts labour at the usual time, so we cannot be exact in discussing the causes of premature labour. Certainly the proper functioning of the placenta is essential to the maintenance of the pregnancy. It is possible that the onset of labour at 40 weeks may be related to the placental ageing which has begun at the 38th week. Possibly premature labour could be due to the placenta working inefficiently at an earlier stage of pregnancy, leading to an early labour, and a live, premature child rather than a death in the uterus. There are, too, women who seem to deliver their young early in every pregnancy, as though it were an individual trait. There seems to be no relation between prematurity and the number of children a woman has, but her age may be a factor. Mothers below twenty years and above forty seem to have a higher prematurity rate than those nearer the middle of their reproductive life.

Sometimes prematurity is caused by surgical intervention on the part of the obstetrician, for some abnormal conditions are treated by the early removal of the infant from the mother's uterus. Pre-eclampsia, with its sharply rising blood pressure, may force the obstetrician to act and to deliver the baby earlier than usual. Sometimes the unborn child is at peril by continuing his intra-uterine existence. The babies of diabetic mothers, for example, are more likely to suffer if left in the uterus after thirty-eight weeks, possibly because of the early ageing of the placenta in such patients. The last chapter showed how the conventional treatment of the Rhesus-affected baby is to remove him from the high concentration of blood antibodies.

More conditions every year are being treated by the early delivery of the baby. This considerably increases the premature baby problem, for, although these infants are being delivered alive, much greater skill and care are required to ensure their continued welfare than are necessary for the more mature child.

Care of the Premature Infant

It is not the purpose of this book to deal with the child after delivery, but several points about the premature baby are relevant. Many babies who weigh just under $5\frac{1}{2}$ pounds enter the category only statistically, and are no different from other children. Those from 4 to 5 pounds should, and infants under 4 pounds must, be admitted to a specialized premature-baby unit. There, trained personnel care for the infant in an incubator, where temperature and humidity control are exact and infection is rigorously excluded. Feeding is difficult at first, and the infant often requires very frequent, small, dilute feeds (see Plate 12).

As in any other branch of medicine, prevention is better than treatment of an established condition. More advances in the treatment of some of the diseases of pregnancy would mean that very early inductions of labour would not be so often forced upon the doctor. Ninety-three per cent of premature labours, however, start spontaneously. Twin pregnancies commonly end early: in Britain the average pair of twins is delivered three weeks before it is due. These twins are small, for, as well as emerging from the uterus short of three weeks' growing time, two babies occupied the place of one. While a single baby born at 37 weeks would weigh about $6\frac{1}{2}$ pounds, twins might weigh only about 5–6 pounds each. Attempts are made to prevent the very premature birth of twins by trying to postpone the normal onset of labour. Mothers with twins are recommended to come into hospital sometime between the 32nd and 36th week of the pregnancy, and here they are strictly rested in bed. This rest sometimes helps to prevent other complications, and the number of very premature labours may be reduced.

Occasionally it is possible to damp down the contractions of the uterus with sedative drugs. If the patient is under surveillance just before labour really starts, heavy sedation can postpone labour. In the research field at present, certain drugs are being elaborated that have a specific effect on the muscle of the uterus. They make the muscle fibres less responsive to stimulation, and so labour can be put off. The group of general sedatives would work only if labour had not really started; once the cervix has started to dilate, very little will stop it. However, the newer muscle relaxants may work even at this later stage, and it would be here that treatment would be most useful, for it is only at this point that most women who are going to deliver prematurely realize they are in labour.

Before we can get further with the problem of preventing prematurity, we must know more about the background of the condition. The size of the mother is important, for a small woman often has a small baby. This child, however, although premature, may not be immature. Certain races, being small in body structure, breed small babies, and this has resulted in the erroneous impression that the Indian women immigrants in Britain have a higher incidence of premature children. The very young mother is twice as likely to have a premature infant as a mother aged more than twenty. Sometimes there is an increased incidence of premature births if the mother has previously had a premature infant. It is interesting that when premature children grow up and marry they do not seem to have any increased tendency to repeat the process: their children often do not come early. Poor feeding, inadequate living accommodation, and bad working conditions are all associated with low economic status, and certainly the risk of prematurity is higher in these groups. In parts of Scotland the incidence of prematurity is twice as high in the lower income groups as in the upper. The former tend to come for ante-natal care later in their pregnancy than do those of higher social classes. Undoubtedly proper attendance at a good clinic can help guard against prematurity, for as well as looking after the patient's diet, the doctor can detect anaemia and make an early diagnosis of pre-eclampsia or of twins.

The Future of the Premature Baby

There are grounds for believing that the human baby is less well adapted for survival in the world than are the young of other animals born after comparable periods of gestation. How much less able to stand the environment is a premature infant. Obviously, the smaller he is, the fewer his chances are. For children born with a weight of about 5 pounds, the infant mortality is about the same as for any other children; from 4 to 5 pounds it is a little higher, but with careful nursing this group often do as well as the heavier babies. Below 4 pounds birth weight, however, mortality levels rise steeply. This is partly owing to the number of congenital abnormalities that occur in this group. Infants with such malformations are often expelled from the uterus early, as is mentioned in Chapters 6 and 7. Premature infants are four times as likely to be born with congenital defects.

Most premature infants now receive care at a proper unit and survive the vicissitudes of early life. Their subsequent progress has been examined by many paediatricians, and compared with that of other children who weighed more than $5\frac{1}{2}$ pounds at birth. An exact comparison is difficult because of the variety of factors associated with the cause of the prematurity. Should the premature infant survive the time of labour and the first weeks of life, then low weight does not seem to interfere with the normal course of development, either physically or mentally. It must be remembered in the first months that the premature baby should be compared with other infants of the same gestational age rather than with those of a similar nominal age. This means that a baby born prematurely at 32 weeks, weighing 4 pounds at birth, should be considered 2 months (eight weeks) behind his nominal age. This difference in actual nominal age is important for comparisons during the first year, but tends to even out by the second or third. Usually infants who are going to be mentally or physically retarded show this in the early months of life. Once the first year is past the infant who is unaffected may be considered as normal as his brothers or sisters of heavier birth weight.

The subsequent progress of premature infants into adult life has been the subject of many myths. Those who become normal children grow into normal adults. It must be remembered that we are all the products of a mass of familial and environmental influences, and that often many of the very causes of a child's prematurity militate against his social and economic future. Most mothers would be proud to have their child grow to become as great a scientist as Charles Darwin, a writer as Victor Hugo, a painter as Renoir or a statesman as Winston Churchill. Yet every one of these men started as a premature baby. Their later lives showed no signs of their small beginnings.

13 | Diseases of the Mother

In Chapter 7, the influence of the mother's health on the very early development of the embryo was considered; now the effects of her ill-health on the whole duration of pregnancy are reviewed. The mother may be suffering from a chronic illness, and pregnancy then occurs as an episode during the period of that ill-health. Alternatively the pregnancy may be in a healthy woman who is attacked by some episode of acute disease. In both groups, the child is normally unaffected. He is well protected, being sheltered by a separate blood supply and buffered by the amniotic fluid around him and the thick muscle of the uterus. Occasionally, however, he is involved in the alterations in the mother's health, and the influence of these on the safety of the unborn child are now examined.

Diabetes

Child-bearing in diabetics is increasing. Years ago it was rare; if diabetic women avoided the risk of early miscarriage, they often lost their babies later in pregnancy or in labour. Diabetes was also formerly often responsible for congenital malformations (dealt with in Chapter 7) owing to an inefficient control of the mother's diabetes and the consequent variations in the balance of her hormones. These risks are greatly reduced in a modern society where ante-natal care ensures that proper attention is paid to the diabetic mother.

When diabetes gets out of control it gives rise to an abnormal usage of the sugar and sugar stores of the body. One of the results of this is the build-up of undesirable chemical side-products when sugar is broken down in the digestive process, so that the concentration of organic compounds (ketones) increases in the mother's blood (ketosis). The fine balance of the body fluids is put out of equilibrium, and a relatively more acid reaction than usual is elicited on testing, for instance, the urine (acidosis). The alterations in the mother's blood are soon reflected in the foetus's blood, and these have harmful effects on the child. To prevent these undesirable biochemical changes very strict control of diabetes must be maintained in pregnancy. Carbohydrate intake and insulin dosage must be finely balanced, and any variations in the blood-sugar levels checked early. In pregnancy there is an increase in the body's rate of usage of carbohydrate, and so the insulin dosage must usually increase in parallel. No fixed rules can be made, for the increase in requirements is not regular: hence the need for the careful checking of diabetes in pregnancy, in order that healthy babies may be produced.

The upset in the mother's hormone state in diabetes is ill understood, but, among the results of the imbalance, a low level of progesterone sometimes occurs. This could influence the tension of the uterine muscle, which may affect the placental blood supply; in an extreme instance this could lead to the premature expulsion of the baby. Lesser degrees of hormone alteration may be responsible for other changes.

The placental bed in the uterus of a diabetic mother has blood vessels which are narrower than in the normal uterus and so less oxygen-rich blood is available for the infant's needs. There is a much greater chance of pre-eclampsia and its attendant risks. Here the raised blood pressure of the mother is related to the poorer blood supply to the infant, and so he is getting still less oxygenated blood.

The babies born of diabetic mothers are much bigger than usual (see Plate 13). The exact reason is not known, but one of the possibilities is that the pituitary gland produces hormone that causes the diabetes. This same substance injected into young animals causes an increase in the growth rate. Possibly, therefore, the growth hormone is the same as the diabetes-producing compound. In the diabetic woman, this compound is circulating in the blood, and when she becomes pregnant it could cross the placenta into the infant. In the mother it is causing a continuance of her diabetes. The infant in the uterus, however, is reacting to it by an increased rate of growth. In addition, the baby is subjected intermittently to swings in the blood-sugar levels. These levels may rise to very high, and act as a short-term stimulus for a temporary speed-up of growth. The infant's resultingly large size often gives rise to difficulties at birth: the poor placental circulation does not allow much margin of safety in the delivery of these babies, and the increased mechanical problem is an added hazard.

For all their size, the babies are often born before their time and are immature. Although they are not premature by the weight definition used in Chapter 12, their organ systems are not fully developed. While a part of the increase in size is due to extra storage of water in the tissues, some is also due to extra growth of the limbs and organs of the body. A proportional increase in the maturation of their function does not occur. It is wise therefore to limit the stresses of labour as much as possible, and to treat the infants of diabetic mothers as 'premature' babies, with the same extra care and nursing skill as the miniature infants receive.

This discussion of the risks to the infant of a diabetic mother may make them seem formidable. Certainly peri-natal mortality is increased in such babies, but careful management of a cooperative mother in the ante-natal period can reduce this. It has, in fact, been lowered consider-ably in the last few years by a firm ante-natal policy run cooperatively by obstetric and diabetic departments. On this cooperation rests the success of the treatment. The sub-sequent description of the management of the pregnancies of diabetic women is based on that carried out at one large hospital in London. There are many variations in the pat-terns of treatment, but this hospital is well known for the excellent results it gets.

Diabetic mothers attend rather more frequently than other mothers at a special ante-natal clinic run by the obstetric and diabetic departments jointly. They are usually main-tained on soluble insulin injections, rather than oral anti-diabetic treatments. Any indications of early infection or pre-eclampsia are dealt with rigorously. At thirty-two weeks, some eight weeks before the expected date of delivery, the mothers are admitted to hospital. Here they have twenty-two hours bed-rest a day, being allowed up for bathing, going to the lavatory and a short spell in a chair. This intensive rest seems hard on an apparently healthy woman, but it serves several functions. Firstly by resting the mother, the energy output is made more constant. A stable output allows greater regulation of food and calorie intake, and this in turn removes one variable in the calculations concerning insulin dosage. Secondly, bed-rest cuts down considerably the incidence of pre-eclampsia and its attendant dangers. Finally, there are some grounds for believing that bed-rest for the mother may allow the infant a better blood supply in the uterus. While the patient is on this regime in hospital, careful watch is kept on her insulin requirements, while the signs of pre-eclampsia – raised blood pressure, swelling of the ankles or protein appearing in the urine – are noted and can be dealt with immediately. The baby in the uterus is examined frequently by palpation, and his heart listened to carefully. If required, X-rays are used to help judge the progress of the infant.

At about the thirty-seventh week, a decision is made in consultation between the obstetrician and the physicians. It is known that placental inefficiency can become manifest in the last two or three weeks of pregnancy, so the time of delivery is planned to avoid this. If the obstetrician thinks that the birth is likely to be a straightforward one with no obvious complications, labour is induced. Should the obstetrical situation be in any way unsatisfactory, then the mother is delivered of the baby by Caesarean section. It is on the skill of choosing which patients are suitable for a vaginal delivery that so much depends.

Delivered, the infant still is at higher risk than normally. He is immature, and all the precautions mentioned in the chapter on prematurity must apply. Once the first week is over he is usually well, having lost much of his excess fluid. Provided they can stand the stresses of delivery and the time immediately following, most infants of diabetic mothers grow up perfectly normally.

Heart Disease

Rheumatic fever is a disease of poor communities. Better housing and feeding have considerably reduced its incidence, and, as a corollary of this, rheumatic heart disease is also on the decline. The total number of pregnant women with congenital heart disease, however, is slightly raised, since advances in heart and chest surgery have rendered more women with congenital heart defects fit for active lives and child-bearing. The overall incidence of all heart disease is, however, falling, and the severity of the condition decreasing.

Pregnancy imposes a load on the heart. Not only is there an increased body weight to which blood must be pumped, but the heart has more blood to deal with and must work harder to achieve the output required. The extra effort required from the heart in the last six months of pregnancy is like that used in walking up a gentle hill. The normal heart can cope with this by compensating mechanisms, but the diseased organ cannot adapt itself so readily and many go into failure. Extra loads besides that due to pregnancy should be avoided. Anaemia, the raised blood pressure of pre-eclampsia, and chest infections are three of these, and a careful watch for them is kept in the ante-natal period.

If the patient is kept well, then the baby develops normally inside the uterus. Any prolonged periods of breathlessness, especially if accompanied by cyanosis, could be hazardous, for the infant too is rendered short of oxygen. Towards the end of pregnancy when the heart begins to get a large volume of blood to deal with, the mother is usually admitted to hospital and rested completely in bed. Delivery must always be in hospital, and a careful watch on the heart's activity is kept during labour. Provided the mother is kept well supplied with oxygen, the baby is perfectly all right at this stage. Labour itself is not usually prolonged in women with heart disease, and the infant is usually born well. As was seen in Chapter 10, he has adaptive mechanisms which enable him to stand slightly lower oxygen levels than the adult.

Tuberculosis

The prevention of pulmonary tuberculosis is one of the greater medical advances in Britain in the last thirty years. The disease is, however, rife in other parts of the world, especially where housing and living standards are poor. Mention has been made, in the chapters on ante-natal care, of the advisability of taking a routine chest X-ray in early pregnancy. In previous years, pregnancy was considered to hasten the progress of tuberculosis and to increase the risk of spreading bacteria. The death rate of infants born to tuberculous mothers was high, for they too contracted the condition. With the newborn's low resistance to infection the chances of cure used to be small.

The discovery of the anti-tuberculosis drugs, streptomycin, para-aminosalicylic acid and isoniazid, has altered this picture. Not only are the numbers of patients greatly reduced, but the disease in any individual can be treated much more effectively now. Should a patient on treatment become pregnant, the drugs being given should be continued. If surgical removal of any tissue is indicated in any special case, it should be undertaken, for it is unlikely that a chest operation will harm the pregnancy. But although these things can be done to help the patient who may have become pregnant while in an active phase of tuberculosis, it is probably wise not to embark deliberately on having a baby at this time. If two or three years can elapse after the disease process has become quiescent, the mother and her baby will benefit.

Through pregnancy, therefore, all treatments that are established are kept going. The position of the anti-tuberculosis drugs in relation to congenital abnormalities is dealt with in Chapter 8. The tubercle bacillus does not cross the placental barrier, and while still unborn the infant is safe from infection. However, once he has been delivered, there is a risk that his mother may infect him by bacilli from her respiratory tract. No closer relationship for the passage of bacteria could be imagined than that of nursing a baby. It is wise, therefore, if the mother has or recently has had 'open tuberculosis' (that is, disease with living bacteria found in her sputum), to isolate the baby from her immediately after birth. This advice sounds harsh, but if it is explained carefully to the mother, it will be accepted as sound sense. No mother would wish actively to infect her baby. She must, however, be warned about the necessity of this separation early in pregnancy. To spring it on her suddenly just after labour would be cruel. When the explanation is given in plenty of time the mother always understands and agrees. The baby is nursed in a special nursery, and when a few days old he is immunized against tuberculosis. After this has been proved by a special skin test (Mantoux reaction) to have been effective, the mother and child may be reunited. The dangers of even a single exposure of the unprotected child to a mother with active tuberculosis cannot be too strongly stressed.

The unborn child is therefore safe from his mother's tuberculosis, and if sensible precautions are taken immediately after birth, he can be kept so.

Syphilis

On her first visit to an ante-natal clinic, every woman has a blood sample taken. A part of this blood is checked by the Wassermann reaction, which detects active syphilis. Most of the mothers in Britain have a negative reaction, but if the disease is present it must be discovered as early as possible in the pregnancy in order to provide adequate treatment for the unborn baby. As well as its tragic effects on the mother's heart, brain and sight, syphilis affects the child in the uterus, even though the maternal infection occurred some time before pregnancy. The more severely affected embryos die and are miscarried, but if the child is less gravely damaged, it may develop to a much later stage in the pregnancy, and then die in the uterus so that a stillbirth follows. A milder degree of involvement allows the baby to be born alive, only to die a few weeks later. Other infants may be born apparently normal and survive. These children may develop the stigmata of syphilis in later childhood and carry through life the bridgeless nose, the deafness, the limp and possibly the cataracts of congenital syphilis. These sequelae can be prevented.

If in early pregnancy the mother is found to have syphilis, treatment is immediately started with large doses of the appropriate antibiotic. When the course is conscientiously taken, the results for the unborn child are excellent; and treatment even at the end of pregnancy is effective in saving the child's life. This venereal disease which formerly caused so much infant death and misery can now be checked, provided proper ante-natal care is given to the mother.

Thyroid Diseases

A goitre is fairly common in women of the age likely to become pregnant. Usually it is of the non-active type, not requiring any treatment unless it obstructs breathing.

Occasionally a more toxic goitre occurs, and a regime of drugs or operations is necessary. If treatment is required during pregnancy, the unborn infant must be considered. If the thyroid gland has been removed by an operation, the woman is probably on a small daily dose of thyroid hormone to keep a natural balance in her body. It is important to assess this correctly. If too little is given, the thyroid gland of the baby in the uterus will become over-active in an effort to supply the mother's body with the hormone. This might lead to an enlargement in the baby's neck that (rarely) causes difficulties in labour. Similarly, too much thyroid extract given to the mother can depress the growth of the baby's gland. This will not show any effects as long as the baby is in the uterus and receiving extra hormone from the mother's blood, but once delivered, he will be thyroid deficient, and weeks might pass before his own gland could make up the arrears.

Some mothers receive drug treatment to suppress the thyroid gland's activity. It must be remembered that a few of these gland depressants cross the placenta and have a similar effect on the baby's thyroid. During pregnancy, such treatment should be carefully supervised by a physician, and only drugs with the least risk used. The infant should be carefully observed after birth so that any signs of thyroid deficiency can be checked. Replacement treatment with thyroid extract can be given, and this corrects the situation.

The five groups of maternal disease considered in this chapter together account for most of the chronic ill-health from which women in the age-group 20–40 may suffer. More rarely, long-term disorders of the nervous system occur; many of these have no effect on the unborn child. Acute infections can also occur and have been discussed in Chapter 7. Women of all age-groups suffer accidents in this fast-moving world; usually, if the mother survives such trauma, the baby in her uterus does too, for he is well protected, being surrounded by numerous built-in defence mechanisms.

No one can help being ill and any woman suffering from the diseases mentioned needs treatment and support. If she becomes pregnant while ill, she owes it to her unborn child to seek help as early as possible from her medical advisers. As has been shown, proper ante-natal care can nearly always lead to an excellent result from the pregnancy.

Outlook

Nature is bountiful, but also wasteful. In the primitive state all species conceive many more progeny than can be allowed to survive into maturity if the ecological balance of living matter is to be kept; when removed from parental influence, vast numbers of these potential offspring die as embryos or infants. Man himself, however, is now in a different position. Since he has made such advances in controlling his environment by far the greater number of his children is likely to survive. The size of the family is therefore generally regulated by means other than fortuitous death after conception. Those children who are born alive are carefully safeguarded.

Resulting from the increased importance accorded to early human life is the need for the greatest possible care of the pregnant mother. Nature's wastefulness is guarded against by the early detection and correction of deviations from the normal. We have come a long way from the 1870s, when ante-natal welfare was first mooted. Then it was for the poor and socially under-privileged, but now almost every pregnant woman in Britain expects that she and her unborn child shall be protected against any possible difficulties in pregnancy.

Most of the women attending ante-natal clinics have no complications, and a normal baby is delivered at the end of pregnancy. With hindsight one might say that their ante-natal attendances were a waste of their and their doctors' time. But this is a dangerous point of view; wisdom after the event is the philosophy of the thoughtless. Only by seeing a woman at regular intervals can her doctor be sure of coping early with potential trouble or, better still, of preventing it. Since the period when ante-natal welfare first began, perinatal mortality has dropped from 153 to 27 per thousand. In this time other factors have also played their part. Better living conditions, advances in medicine and more deliveries in hospital certainly have reduced the numbers of infant deaths; the ante-natal clinic still stands as one of the best examples of preventive medicine. To maintain this improved state demands constant watch by the obstetrician and repeated visits by the patient. Only so will we reduce the wastage still more. Regular attendance at her ante-natal clinic is the most important contribution any mother can make to the safety of her unborn child.

Chronological Table

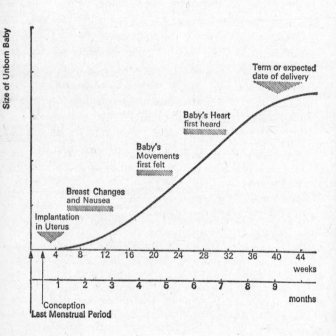

Glossary

Abdomen: The medical term for the lower trunk between the diaphragm and the pelvis. Colloquially, it is the belly. The more refined 'stomach' is less correct, for this strictly refers to only one organ inside the abdomen.

Abortion: The expulsion of a foetus before the 28th week of pregnancy. This may be spontaneous or induced. The medical man uses the term abortion for both situations; the general public keep it for the second, while the first they call a miscarriage.

Acidosis: The accumulation of ketonse (q.v.) and other acidic products in the body when the balance of the internal chemistry becomes disturbed. These substances can be detected in the blood and urine of such patients and the balance corrected by appropriate treatment. Acidosis can arise in the course of a long labour or in diabetes.

Adrenal Glands: A complex pair of endocrine glands (q.v.) placed just above the kidneys. They make hormones that affect all bodily functions and are principally concerned in helping to keep the internal environment of the body constant.

Anoxia: A state in which the body is deprived of oxygen. Strictly anoxia means no oxygen, a biological situation that is almost impossible to achieve. The term anoxia is commonly used for low oxygen situations, when perhaps the word hypoxia would be better.

Antibiotic: A substance obtained from a fungus, which destroys or inhibits the growth of micro-organisms. The first to be discovered was penicillin. About thirty others have since been used in medicine.

Antibody: A product of the body's reaction to an outside influence. Should a foreign protein get into the body, the cells make antibodies which will destroy the protein.

Blood Sugar: The amount of sugar in the blood. Among the foodstuffs dissolved in the circulating blood is glucose. This can be accurately measured in a drop of blood from the finger or the ear and represents the levels in the body. The concentrations vary greatly in relation to eating; in hunger they are low, after eating they are high.

Cell: The smallest unit of biological life. All tissues in plants and

177

animals are composed of these minute 'bricks'. They are very small and can be examined only through a microscope. Their size can be gauged from the fact that a teaspoonful of blood would contain two thousand million red-blood cells.

Cervix: The lowest part of the uterus, that part which acts as the neck of the organ. This neck dilates in labour to allow the passage of the baby's head.

Conception: The fusing of the egg with the sperm, and thus the start of the new individual. Since it takes place inside the mother's body, we use the active verb in connexion with her only ('The woman conceived and brought forth a son').

Control: A statistical term meaning anything that can be used as a standard for checking observations. When an experiment is performed, many of the variable factors are guarded against by the use of controls. Perhaps a drug is being tested on animals by injection. Then a similar batch of animals is used as a control for the experimental group. The control animals are given an injection of simple salt water, but otherwise share the same conditions as the tested group. Any difference of reaction between the two groups can then legitimately be supposed to be due to the injected drug.

Cyanosis: A condition in which the blood contains less oxygen than normal, which gives the blood, and hence the skin, a bluish tinge. The lesser degrees are first seen at the lips and finger-nails; later the face and hands are involved.

Diabetes: A metabolic disease which affects the function of the liver and pancreas. The body's ability to deal with glucose is impaired and so great fluctuations of blood sugar (q.v.) occur. Sugar can be detected in the urine. The condition can be treated by insulin (q.v.), which helps to stabilize the utilization of sugar.

Dominance: In discussing inherited characteristics some genes are considered dominant over others (which are called recessive). The dominant genes will always pass on the traits they carry to all offspring; the recessive gene will do so only if paired with another recessive gene.

Down's Syndrome: A new name for what was called mongolism. It is a form of mental defect; details are given in Chapter 7.

Ectopic Pregnancy: A pregnancy in the wrong place. All normal pregnancies occur in the cavity of the uterus. Rarely the egg settles elsewhere; this may be in one of the Fallopian tubes in which case its continued growth may go on to tear this narrow structure.

Electrocardiography: A method of detecting, amplifying and recording the electrical activity of the heart.

Embryo: A developing human baby in the first eight weeks of its intra-uterine existence, during which stage the organs are being formed. After the eighth week it is called a foetus (q.v.), and its further intra-uterine progress is by growth of the structures already formed, rather than by initiation of anything new.

Engagement: As applied to a baby this means that the biggest diameter of the infant's head has entered the mother's pelvis. It often happens in the last two or three weeks of the first pregnancy, but may not occur until the onset of labour in later deliveries.

Enzymes: Chemicals existing in cells which speed up reactions, such as the utilization of oxygen and the break-down of energy-rich food-stuffs.

Foetus: A developing human baby for the last 32 weeks of intra-uterine life. During this period it is developing the organ structures laid down in the earlier (embryonic) part of its existence.

It is probably more correct to spell this word fetus as the Americans do. However, in this book we have retained the older and more familiar spelling.

Gland: An anatomical term meaning an organ (q.v.) that secretes. Glands are of two sorts: (1) those that secrete to the outside, as for example the breast secretes milk and the sweat glands secrete sweat; (2) those that secrete into the blood stream, for example the pituitary gland and the thyroid gland. The second group are called endocrine glands and make hormones (q.v.).

Gravid: Pregnant. From the Latin, *gravidus.*

Haemoglobin: The iron pigment in the blood that carries oxygen to all the tissues.

Heterozygous: A term used in genetics, implying that the two genes determining a single characteristic in the chromosomes of the person involved are unlike. Consequently, in the splitting of the chromosomes for the formation of the sex cells, dissimilar genes are carried in the sperm or ovum, allowing of a greater variety of inherited characteristics than would be possible where the genes were identical. (see below.)

Homozygous: The opposite of heterozygous. In these cases all the sperm or all the ova carry identical genes for a particular characteristic, so that in this respect all offspring inherit the same factor from the parent.

Glossary

Hormones: Hormones act as the chemical messengers in the blood stimulating the body's cells to perform their functions. They are produced by the endocrine glands (q.v.), and they influence such things as growth, water balance, metabolism, temperature control and secondary sex characteristics.

Hydrocephalus: A condition of 'water on the brain' in the infant. It is normal to have fluid bathing the nervous system, but in hydrocephaly the fluid is in excess. All degrees exist, from the mildest cases that are recognizable only on special X-rays to those immediately obvious from the size of the head. Infants with a serious degree of hydrocephaly have great difficulty at delivery. The milder cases respond well to special treatments that can be given in specialist paediatric departments.

Hypoglycaemia: A condition of abnormally low sugar content in the blood. If the level drops too low the patient feels faint.

Immature: An immature infant is one who is not fully developed. He is often premature (q.v.) and may have been delivered before he was due. His organ systems are less capable of dealing with stress, and have not achieved their full functional capacity.

Insulin: A chemical similar to an extract from the tissues of the pancreas, which is given by injection in the treatment of diabetes (q.v.). It helps to stabilize the fluctuations of blood sugar that occur in diabetes.

Irradiation: The exposure of tissues to X-rays. Every time a diagnostic X-ray is taken, a very small amount of irradiation occurs. The situation as regards pregnancy is fully discussed in Chapter 7.

Isotope: All elements have an atomic number which bears a relation to their chemical properties. However, each individual element may have a number of forms which contain different numbers of electrons. Chemically these forms (isotopes) all act in the same fashion. Physically, however, they are different and often are unstable and radioactive. For example, iodine is usually formed as the isotope I_{126}; further isotopes, I_{125}, I_{131} and I_{132}, can be made and are all radioactive.

Ketones and Ketosis: Ketones are some of the waste products of the body which collect in abnormally large quantities in the blood and urine of persons suffering from acidosis (q.v.). A patient in whom these ketones are detected is said to be suffering from ketosis. This condition occasionally arises after some unusually hard physical effort (for example, labour).

Labour: Labour is the forceful contractions of the uterus which end in the delivery of the baby. It is of variable duration, usually being longer for the first child than for subsequent infants. Labour rarely lasts more than thirty hours; usually it is over in twenty-four.

Lymph Nodes: Small collections of tissue scattered throughout the body, which act as filters for lymph, the nutrient fluid which bathes all the body tissues. In certain infections these nodes become enlarged and tender owing to the presence of large numbers of bacteria and cells concerned with the body's defensive mechanism.

Mantoux Test: A test for susceptibility to tuberculosis. A minute quantity of killed tubercle bacilli is scratched into the skin. If the subject has previously had a tuberculous infection, he will have formed antibodies which will remain in his blood stream, and a mild reaction will appear at the site of the scratch. This is considered as a positive Mantoux reaction, showing that the subject is immune to further infection by the tubercle bacillus. The vast majority of town-dwellers in Britain have been exposed to minute doses of tuberculosis in early youth and have a positive Mantoux reaction.

Maturity: In pregnancy, this refers to the stage the intra-uterine baby has reached. Pregnancy usually lasts 280 days or 40 weeks (see Chapter 2).

Membrane: A thin layer of tissue surrounding every cell (q.v.) in the body which allows the diffusion of oxygen and foodstuffs.

Molecule: This is the smallest quantity of any chemical which can exist. It is composed of the actual atoms that make up the compound. So small are molecules that most of them can pass through membranes by diffusion.

Mongolism: An old-fashioned name for a condition of infant mental retardation now called Down's syndrome (see Chapter 7).

Neonatal: An adjective applied to newborn babies. They are in the neonatal period until they are a month old. After this they are called infants and, after a year, children.

Nucleus: That part of the cell which controls its activity. It is the area in which all the chromosome material is stored and so all the genetic potentials exist here.

Organ: This anatomical term is applied to any part of the body that is characterized by a particular function. The eye, the stomach and the uterus, for example, are made up of different types of tissues, but each group of tissues is geared to a separate function – respectively seeing, digesting or child-bearing.

Glossary

Perinatal: An adjective to describe the period of time that includes late pregnancy and the first week after delivery. Thus perinatal mortality indicates the deaths of babies in the last twelve weeks of pregnancy and the first week after birth.

Phocomelia: The condition of being born with stunted limbs. The hands, or feet, spring straight from the trunk. This is an exceedingly rare abnormality; it occurred after Thalidomide was taken by mothers in the early weeks of pregnancy.

Pituitary Gland: An endocrine gland in the brain. It makes hormones that control the function of all the other internal glands of the body. The pituitary is rightly called 'the conductor of the endocrine orchestra'.

Placenta: A disc of tissue, closely adherent to the uterine wall, connected by arteries and a vein with the embryonic circulation. Here oxygen and foodstuffs diffuse into, and waste products leave, the infant's circulation. After delivery, it is no longer required and is expelled. It is popularly known as the 'afterbirth'.

Plasma: The fluid part of mammalian blood: consists of millions of red and white cells suspended in this fluid. Plasma is what remains if the cells are filtered off. It contains proteins and other foodstuffs, antibodies and small traces of hormones and salts.

Pre-eclampsia: A condition, arising only in pregnancy, where the blood pressure is raised and there is an accumulation of fluid in the body tissues, making them puffy. The kidney's function is also altered, so that a little of the blood's protein leaks into the urine. This condition used to be very serious for the mother for it could lead to eclampsia, in which fits may occur. However, modern ante-natal care has lowered this risk, and patients are carefully checked for the earliest signs of pre-eclampsia. Vigorous treatment at this stage prevents the more serious sequelae.

Premature: A premature infant is one that weighs less than 5½ pounds. This is an international definition.

Rhesus Factor: The blood of 85 per cent of humans contains an agglutinating factor similar to that found in the Rhesus monkey. If it is present, the person is Rhesus positive; if absent, Rhesus negative.

Rubella: A virus infection causing a mild illness (German measles). Although the adult is not seriously ill, the unborn child may be affected if the illness occurs during early pregnancy (Chapter 7).

Sedative: A medicine that quietens a patient or decreases excitement.

Often such treatment is prescribed to help those who cannot sleep at night. It is also used to prevent the rise of blood pressure in the treatment of pre-eclampsia.

Serum: A portion of the fluid part of the blood. Blood consists of cells suspended in plasma (q.v.). One of the major proteins dissolved in plasma is concerned with clotting (fibrinogen). Once this protein is removed, the plasma cannot clot and serum remains. Thus serum contains all the valuable constituents of plasma other than the clotting protein.

Sonar: Sound waves can be reflected from hard objects, and when this takes place in the air the phenomenon is called an echo. Similarly, sound waves can be transmitted through solid materials and their reflections recorded. Calculations can be made of the distances involved and so a 'picture' of the reflecting echoes can be built up. In Chapter 3 the use of Sonar in plotting the shape and position of the unborn baby is discussed.

Spina Bifida: Split spine. Occasionally, the spinal bones are not properly fused. Then the sac of membrane covering the spinal cord bulges out (meningoceole); sometimes the cord itself is protruded also in the sac (meningomyelocoele).

Steroid: A chemical with a complex chemical formula: many of the hormones (q.v.) in the body have this chemical structure, as for instance those made by the adrenal glands and the ovaries.

Stillbirth: A baby that is born dead. The legal definition lays down that the pregnancy must have passed 28 weeks and that the baby showed no signs of life after leaving the mother.

Syndrome: A medical term meaning a collection of symptoms. It has a looser meaning than the word disease but covers a similar context.

Syphilis: A venereal disease transmitted from the sexual organs of one person to another. If untreated it has permanent serious effects on the health of a woman, affecting her heart and brain; and should she become pregnant, the unborn child might also be affected. Proper treatment in pregnancy can prevent this happening.

Teratogenesis: The capacity to alter normal intra-uterine development and so cause malformations.

Term: The time when a pregnant woman might expect her baby to be born. Term is usually 280 days or 40 weeks after the first day of the last menstrual period.

Thalidomide: A sedative drug used in the 1950s, and thought at the time to be perfectly safe. Unfortunately it had one side effect – it damaged embryos at a critical stage in their development. It is not now used. Its effects are dealt with in Chapter 8.

Thyroid Gland: An endocrine gland (q.v.) in the neck. It makes a hormone (thyroxine) that affects the rate of bodily activity.

Thyrotoxicosis: A disease of the thyroid gland (q.v.) which is characterized by over-production of the thyroid hormone. This makes the patient nervous and hyper-excitable.

Toxaemia: See Pre-eclampsia.

Tuberculosis: A chest infection which used to kill (Mimi in *La Bohème* dies dramatically from it). Now modern drugs have taken away many of the dangers. It is caused by bacteria that spread in the cough of affected people. The Mass Miniature X-ray service has reduced the amount of tuberculosis by early diagnosis which ensures for such patients early treatment.

Villus: A projection of tissue from the foetal side of the placenta, which is bathed by the mother's blood. Through the cell membranes of the villus food and oxygen can pass from the mother to the unborn child.

Virus: A very small infective agent. Diseases are carried by viruses, which are much smaller than bacteria.

Wassermann Reaction: A blood test for syphilis (q.v.) (see Chapter 13).

X-rays: Invisible rays that can penetrate tissues. Harder structures reflect X-rays best, and so bones show up easily on photographic films exposed. By means of these rays, the baby can be viewed in the mother's abdomen from twenty weeks onwards.

More about Penguins and Pelicans

Penguinews, which appears every month, contains details
of all the new books issued by Penguins as they are
published. From time to time it is supplemented by
Penguins in Print – a complete list of all our available titles.
(There are well over three thousand of these.)

A specimen copy of *Penguinews* will be sent to you free on
request, and you can become a subscriber for the price of the
postage – 4s. for a year's issues (including the complete
lists). Just write to Dept EP, Penguin Books Ltd,
Harmondsworth, Middlesex, enclosing a cheque or
postal order, and your name will be added to the
mailing list.

Some other books published by Penguins are
described on the following pages.

Note: *Penguinews* and *Penguins in Print*
are not available in the U.S.A. or Canada

Patterns of Infant Care in an Urban Community

John and Elizabeth Newson

Mother, doctor, health visitor, midwife – Spock, Gibbens, de Kok, Truby King ... the amount of theory and advice, both professional and amateur, that showers on the young mother is equalled only by its astonishing contradictions. And indeed, as the authors quietly point out, 'very few theories of child rearing have been subjected to the inconvenience of being reconciled with the empirical evidence'.

What then is that evidence? Armed with common sense and a tape recorder, the authors interviewed in their Nottingham homes over 700 mothers of one-year-old children to find out, quite simply, how babies are brought up in England today. The result is a landmark in our knowledge of childhood. The answers parents gave on subjects ranging from breast- and bottle-feeding, sleeping, eating, and punishment, to father's place in the home and class differences in infant rearing make a fascinating and, on occasions, hilarious kaleidoscope of life with young children.

'Wonderfully human piece of sociological research' – *Yorkshire Post*

Child Care and the Growth of Love

New Enlarged Edition

John Bowlby

In 1951, under the auspices of the World Health
Organization, Dr John Bowlby wrote a report on *Maternal
Care and Mental Health* which collated expert world opinion
on the subject and the issues arising from it – the prevention
of juvenile and adult delinquency, the problem of the
'unwanted child', the training of women for motherhood,
and the best ways of supplying the needs of children
deprived of their natural mothers. This book is a summary
of Dr Bowlby's report, freed from many of its technicalities
and prepared for the general reader.

This new edition contains chapters based on an article
by Dr Mary Salter Ainsworth, written in 1962 also for the
World Health Organization when it once again made an
important study of child care.

'It is a convenient and scholarly summary of evidence of
the effects upon children of lack of personal attention, and
it presents to administrators, social workers, teachers and
doctors a reminder of the significance of the family' –
The Times

The Experience of Childbirth

Sheila Kitzinger

'For far too many women pregnancy and birth is still something that happens to them rather than something they set out consciously and joyfully to do themselves.'

The Experience of Childbirth is written by a sociologist and ante-natal teacher – herself the mother of five children – as a complete manual of physical and emotional preparation for the expectant mother. The physiology of pregnancy, the development of the foetus, and the successive stages of labour are described in detail. Moving on from the pioneer work of Grantly Dick-Read and later psychoprophylactic techniques Mrs Kitzinger's research and teaching focus particularly on the psychological aspects of child-bearing, on the preparation of both wife and husband not only for birth but for parenthood and marital adjustment, and on a girl's changing relationship with her own mother.

Mrs Kitzinger has completely re-written her book for this Pelican edition, developing new breathing and relaxation techniques to help maintain control in labour. One section is addressed to prospective fathers, another to prospective grandmothers, and she has added many personal accounts of labour recorded by some of the hundreds of women who have been her pupils.

Not for sale in the U.S.A.

A Penguin Handbook

Childbirth

W. C. W. Nixon

The author of this informative handbook is Professor of
Obstetrics and Gynaecology in the University of London
and has been director of the obstetric unit at University
College Hospital since 1946.

'With every advance, scientific or sociological,' he
writes, 'the hazards of childbirth are being still further
reduced. Yet there are a number of women who fear
pregnancy and labour . . . I believe, through personal
observation, that one can face a situation much better if
one knows the facts. The purpose of this book is to
present some of the facts which have an important bearing
on the process of birth.' This helpful account of what can
be the happiest experience in a woman's life is well
illustrated with diagrams (of exercises) and plates of a
remarkable series of models.